BLOOD SUGAR DIET SOLUTION

A comprehensive guide to initiating a successful blood sugar diet transformation with a systematic approach

MONICA EDWARD

TABLE OF CONTENT

BLOOD SUGAR DIET SOLUTION

Chapter 10: Long-Term Maintenance and Support
Strategies for Maintaining Blood Sugar Stability
Seeking Professional Guidance and Support

Conclusion
Achieving Balanced Blood Sugar and Improved
Wellbeing

Introduction

Once upon a time, in a small town nestled among rolling hills, there lived a man named Thomas. Thomas was a kind and observant person who had a lifelong fascination with the mysteries of the human body. He had a passion for studying health and nutrition and an insatiable hunger for knowledge.

One day, as Thomas was browsing through the dusty shelves of a local bookstore, he stumbled upon an old, leather-bound book with golden inscriptions that read "The Secrets of Optimal Health." Intrigued, he took it in his hands and gently blew off the accumulated dust, revealing its title. Excitement welled up inside him, and he felt as though he had stumbled upon a treasure trove of wisdom.

As he thumbed through the pages, his eyes fell upon a chapter titled "The Hidden Power of Blood Sugar." His heart raced with anticipation, sensing he had found something truly special.
The chapter detailed the profound impact blood sugar levels have on a person's health and how imbalances could lead to numerous complications and diseases. Thomas studied the book for hours every day, determined to discover the secrets that lay within. Managing blood sugar levels could be key to preventing and treating a number of medical conditions, according

to a theory that captivated him. He buried himself in research papers, medical journals, and countless scientific studies, consumed by zeal and infatuation.

Days turned into weeks, and weeks turned into months. Thomas's eyes grew tired, but his determination remained unwavering. Finally, after months of tireless dedication, he emerged triumphant. He had created a revolutionary blood sugar diet solution that could be transformative for individuals struggling with diabetes, obesity, and other related ailments.

Thomas named his programme "Glycen," derived from the Greek word "glykys," meaning sweet, symbolizing the need to control the sweetness that floods through our veins. Excited to share his discovery with the world, he set up a small clinic in his town, offering seminars and assistance to those in need.

Word of his amazing achievement spread like wildfire, reaching far beyond the borders of his small town. People traveled from near and far, seeking Thomas's guidance and hoping for a chance to turn their lives around. The success stories piled up—individuals who once suffered endlessly from fatigue, weight gain, and high blood sugar levels experienced newfound vitality and control over their health.

As his reputation grew, Thomas received numerous invitations to speak at international conferences and

prestigious institutes. He stood on stage, sharing his story and knowledge, inspiring others to take charge of their health just as he had. Scientists and doctors marvelled at his innovation, and he became a beacon of hope for those longing for a better life.
With every passing year, Thomas's influence expanded further. His revolutionary Glycen programme spread across the globe, helping countless individuals regain control over their blood sugar levels and transform their overall health. His book was translated into many languages and went on to become a best-seller, furthering his legacy of enhancing people's lives.

Thomas had unwittingly become the hero of a story he never knew he would write. Through his insatiable curiosity, dedication, and unwavering belief in the power of knowledge, he forever changed the lives of countless individuals. As he looked back at the path he had walked, he couldn't help but feel grateful for the day he stumbled upon that dusty, old book, unlocking a secret that would change the world.
Rebalance Your Blood Sugar: The Ultimate Guide to Better Health.

Chapter 1:
Understanding Blood Sugar and its Impact on Health

Getting started with a blood sugar diet solution is a proactive and successful method for regulating blood sugar levels and improving overall health. A blood sugar diet solution focuses on managing blood sugar levels through balanced and healthy meals, lifestyle adjustments, and frequent physical activity. This thorough content will walk you through the important parts of establishing a blood sugar diet plan.

Understanding the Blood Sugar Diet Solution:

The blood sugar diet approach is based on an understanding of how specific foods affect blood sugar levels. It emphasizes including low-glycemic index (GI) items in your diet, which helps stabilize blood sugar levels and prevent spikes and crashes.

Whole grains, legumes, lean meats, healthy fats, and fiber-rich fruits and vegetables are examples of these foods.

Consultation with a Healthcare Professional:
Before beginning any diet or lifestyle modification, it is critical to check with a healthcare expert, especially if you have diabetes or another medical condition. They can give you specific advice depending on your health status, medications, and nutritional needs.

Establishing Specific Objectives:
Determine the objectives you wish to achieve with the blood sugar diet strategy. Whether you want to lose weight, manage diabetes, increase energy, or improve your general health, establishing clear goals will help you stay motivated and stick to your diet plan.

Educating yourself:
Learn about carbs, the glycemic index, portion control, and reading food labels, among other aspects of blood sugar management. Understanding how different foods affect your blood sugar levels allows you to make more informed decisions.

Creating a Well-Balanced Meal Plan:
Create a meal plan that incorporates a range of low-GI meals while also ensuring a balance of macronutrients—carbohydrates, proteins, and fats.
This balance helps to control blood sugar levels, keep you full, and sustain energy levels throughout the day.

Include entire grains, legumes, lean meats, fatty fish, nuts, seeds, healthy oils, and plenty of veggies and fruits.

Including regular physical activity:
Physical activity is critical for blood sugar management. Regular exercise improves insulin sensitivity, weight control, and overall fitness. Walk, swim, cycle, or dance for at least 150 minutes every week.

Practicing Portion Control:
When it comes to controlling blood sugar levels, portion control is essential. Consume smaller, more regular meals rather than large, infrequent ones to avoid blood sugar rises. To promote satiety, use smaller dishes and whole grains instead of processed grains.

Stress Management and Sleep:
Stress and a lack of sleep can have a major impact on blood sugar levels. Incorporate stress-management practices such as meditation, deep breathing exercises, and hobbies. Aim for 7-9 hours of excellent sleep per night to maintain appropriate blood sugar management.

Monitoring blood sugar levels:
Monitor your blood sugar levels with a glucometer regularly to determine the impact of your dietary and lifestyle adjustments. This will aid in identifying any

necessary changes to your strategy and allow for better blood sugar management.

Seeking Assistance:
Consider joining support groups, internet forums, or receiving advice from a licensed dietitian specializing in blood sugar management. Sharing experiences, struggles, and success stories with others on a similar journey can bring motivation and encouragement.

To summarize, starting a blood sugar diet solution includes understanding the impact of food choices on blood sugar levels, planning well-balanced meal plans, adding regular physical activity, managing stress and sleep, and monitoring blood sugar levels. By applying these measures, you can effectively regulate your blood sugar levels, improve your general health, and improve your quality of life.

The Basics of Blood Sugar

Blood sugar, often known as blood glucose, is the amount of sugar (glucose) in the blood. It is the principal source of energy for the cells in our bodies and is essential for overall health. Understanding the fundamentals of blood sugar is critical for managing and preventing a variety of health problems, including diabetes.

Glucose is derived from meals and delivered through the bloodstream to many organs and cells in the body. The pancreas produces two hormones that govern this process: insulin and glucagon. Insulin facilitates the entry of glucose into cells, where it is transformed into energy or stored for later use. Glucagon, on the other hand, helps to raise blood sugar levels when they are too low.

The typical blood sugar level fluctuates depending on several factors, including an individual's age, time of day, and whether or not they have recently eaten. However, the typical range for fasting blood sugar is between 70 and 99 mg/dL (3.9 and 5.5 mmol/L). Blood sugar levels normally rise after a meal but should return to normal within a few hours. Elevated or low blood sugar levels can signal underlying health issues or insulin production and usage abnormalities.

High blood sugar, often known as hyperglycemia, happens when the body does not create enough insulin or is unable to use the insulin that it does make adequately. Individuals with diabetes or prediabetes may experience this. Prolonged high blood sugar levels can cause difficulties and damage to organs such as the eyes, kidneys, nerves, and heart. Hyperglycemia symptoms include excessive thirst, frequent urination, weariness, impaired vision, and poor wound healing.

Low blood sugar, also known as hypoglycemia, is more likely in diabetics who use insulin or other blood sugar-lowering drugs. It can also develop in people who do not have diabetes as a result of heavy alcohol consumption, certain drugs, or prolonged fasting. If left untreated, hypoglycemia symptoms can include shakiness, perspiration, rapid heartbeat, confusion, and even loss of consciousness.

A balanced lifestyle is vital for maintaining good blood sugar levels. This involves eating nutritious food, exercising regularly, maintaining a healthy weight, and managing stress.
A diet high in whole grains, fruits and vegetables, lean meats, and healthy fats can help keep blood sugar levels stable.
Avoiding high-sugar and processed foods is critical because they promote blood sugar spikes and crashes. Monitoring blood sugar levels is critical for diabetics to avoid complications. This is usually accomplished through regular blood sugar testing using a glucose monitor. Based on these findings, suitable adjustments to medication, diet, and lifestyle choices can be made to keep blood sugar levels within the desired range.

In conclusion, blood sugar levels are critical to general health. Understanding the fundamentals of blood sugar, such as the normal range, causes and symptoms of high and low blood sugar, and lifestyle measures to regulate it, is critical for preventing and managing diseases such as diabetes. Individuals can maintain maximum health and well-being by adopting a balanced lifestyle and routinely monitoring blood sugar levels.

The Role of Blood Sugar in Metabolism:

Blood Sugar's Role in Metabolism
The process by which the body turns food and drink into energy is known as metabolism.
It entails a series of chemical events that take place within cells, allowing the body to break down foods like carbs, lipids, and proteins and transform them into useful energy.
Blood sugar, commonly known as blood glucose, is an important component that influences metabolism.
Blood sugar is the glucose present in the bloodstream and is the body's principal source of energy. Glucose is obtained from the digestion and breakdown of carbohydrates in our diet. Once absorbed into the bloodstream, it is carried to cells throughout the body and used as fuel to perform numerous bodily activities. Blood sugar control is critical for sustaining good metabolic function. The body has a sophisticated system in place to control blood sugar levels within a limited range, which is usually between 70 and 110 milligrammes per deciliter (mg/dL). The pancreas, liver,

and hormones such as insulin and glucagon are all important participants in this system.

Insulin, a hormone produced by the pancreatic beta cells, plays a major role in controlling blood sugar levels. The pancreas produces insulin in the bloodstream when blood sugar levels rise after a meal. Insulin functions like a key, allowing glucose to enter and be used as energy. It also instructs the liver to store excess glucose as glycogen for later use.
Thus, low insulin levels or insulin resistance can result in hyperglycemia or high blood sugar levels. High insulin levels, on the other hand, can drop blood sugar levels, resulting in hypoglycemia. Hyperglycemia and hypoglycemia can both have serious consequences for metabolism and general health.

The body uses glucose as its principal source of energy in a healthy metabolic system. During periods of fasting or high energy demands, the body may need to access stored glucose sources, such as glycogen in the liver.
The pancreas generates another hormone called glucagon in response to decreasing blood sugar levels.
Glucagon instructs the liver to degrade glycogen and release glucose into the bloodstream, providing the body with an easily accessible source of energy.

Furthermore, blood sugar levels affect the metabolism of other nutrients, such as fats and proteins. When blood sugar levels are low, the body may turn to fat for energy via a process known as lipolysis. Lipolysis is the breakdown of stored fat into fatty acids, which cells can use as an alternative energy source. Chronically high blood sugar levels, on the other hand, can disrupt this process and encourage fat formation.

Furthermore, blood sugar levels are important for appetite management.

High blood sugar levels can cause the production of hormones such as leptin, which indicates fullness and aids in the regulation of food consumption. Low blood sugar levels, on the other hand, can cause the production of ghrelin, a hunger-stimulating hormone. Blood sugar imbalances might interfere with these hunger and satiety signals, potentially leading to overeating or increased food cravings.

In conclusion, blood sugar levels are critical to overall metabolic activity. Blood sugar control ensures that the body has a steady and stable supply of energy. Blood sugar regulation disruptions, whether caused by insulin resistance, diabetes, or other reasons, can have far-reaching consequences for metabolism, hunger regulation, and overall health. Maintaining appropriate blood sugar levels through a well-balanced diet, frequent physical activity, and proper medical care is therefore critical for good metabolic function.

Health Implications of Imbalanced Blood Sugar Levels,

Blood sugar imbalances, also known as blood glucose levels, can have serious health consequences and are frequently linked to a variety of medical disorders. The amount of glucose present in the bloodstream is referred to as blood sugar, and it is an important source of energy for the body's cells. When blood sugar levels are out of balance, either too high (hyperglycemia) or too low (hypoglycemia), the effects on overall health and well-being can be severe.

Let us investigate the health consequences of these scenarios.

Diabetes:

When blood sugar levels are increased, hyperglycemia ensues. Ineffective insulin use by the body or a shortage of insulin are the common causes of this. Here are the health consequences of high blood sugar levels:

Type 2 diabetes is characterized by insulin resistance, resulting in persistent hyperglycemia. Diabetes can cause damage to different organs and systems over time, increasing the risk of cardiovascular disease, stroke, renal disease, visual issues, and nerve damage.

Metabolic syndrome: High blood sugar levels regularly can lead to metabolic syndrome, a group of disorders that includes obesity, high blood pressure, high cholesterol, and insulin resistance. This combination increases the risk of cardiovascular disease, stroke, and type 2 diabetes considerably.

Increased infection risk: Because hyperglycemia affects the immune system, people are more prone to infections, particularly in the urinary tract, skin, and oral cavity. It also slows wound healing, putting diabetics at risk of infection.

Diabetic ketoacidosis (DKA): When blood sugar levels rise to dangerously high levels, patients with type 1 diabetes may develop DKA, a potentially fatal illness in which the body produces ketones as an alternative fuel source, resulting in acidosis, dehydration, and organ damage.

Hyperglycemia:
Hypoglycemia occurs when blood sugar levels fall below normal, which can happen as a result of too much insulin, a poor diet, or certain drugs. Low blood sugar levels can have the following health consequences: Inadequate glucose delivery to the brain can induce disorientation, difficulty concentrating, irritability, and dizziness. Seizures, loss of consciousness, and coma can result from severe and sustained hypoglycemia.

Enhanced cardiovascular risks: Hypoglycemia can cause irregular heartbeats, palpitations, and, in severe situations, heart attacks. It makes people more susceptible to cardiovascular issues, especially those who already have heart disease.

Low blood sugar levels can cause exhaustion, weakness, shakiness, and a lack of vitality. This can have an impact on physical performance as well as daily routines. Hypoglycemia can cause anxiety, mood fluctuations, irritation, and feelings of discomfort. The anxiety of hypoglycemia episodes in diabetics can cause psychological stress and negatively impair their emotional well-being.

A balanced diet, frequent physical activity, medication (if necessary), and a healthy lifestyle are essential for controlling blood sugar levels.

Blood glucose levels should be checked regularly, especially for people who have diabetes or are at risk of developing it. Maintaining stable blood sugar levels is critical for overall health and can greatly lower the risk of problems.

Chapter 2:
The Blood Sugar Diet Solution:
An Overview

The Blood Sugar Diet Solution is a complete and successful method for controlling blood sugar levels and losing weight. This diet plan was created by British TV journalist and physician Dr. Michael Mosley, and it claims to improve general health, facilitate long-term weight loss, and prevent and reverse type 2 diabetes.

The Blood Sugar Diet Solution, at its foundation, stresses the eating of low-carbohydrate, nutrient-dense foods while limiting the consumption of high-sugar and high-carb choices. The major goal is to regulate blood sugar levels by eating healthily and following an intermittent fasting schedule.

One of the major ideas of this diet is the "800-calorie diet," in which participants consume around 800 calories per day for a certain length of time. This low-calorie phase lasts for 8 weeks and is thought to kickstart weight reduction, reduce inflammation, and enhance insulin sensitivity.

Individuals typically consume low-carb veggies, lean proteins, healthy fats, and a limited amount of low-sugar fruits during this phase. These foods are known to supply critical nutrients, keep you satiated, and keep your blood sugar levels stable.

Intermittent fasting is another important part of the blood sugar diet. Participants engage in alternate-day fasting or time-restricted eating, which limits their eating window to a certain number of hours per day. Allowing the body to enter a fasting state allows it to burn stored fat while maintaining appropriate blood sugar levels. The Blood Sugar Diet Solution strongly encourages regular physical activity.

Exercise not only helps with weight loss, but it also helps with insulin sensitivity, blood sugar regulation, and general cardiovascular health.

Following the Blood Sugar Diet Solution has resulted in many favorable effects. They have lost weight, reduced their cravings for sugary meals, increased their energy levels, and improved their blood sugar management. It is crucial to note, however, that individual results may vary, and the food plan should be tailored to individual needs and health situations.

To summarize, the Blood Sugar Diet Solution provides a comprehensive and long-term method for controlling blood sugar levels and losing weight. Individuals can not only avoid or reverse type 2 diabetes by focusing on nutrient-dense diets, intermittent fasting, and regular exercise, but they can also enhance general health and well-being.

What is a blood sugar diet?

A blood sugar diet, also known as a low-glycemic index (GI) diet, is a nutritional approach that aims to regulate and stabilize blood sugar levels. It focuses on eating foods with a lower GI rating, which promotes a slower and more steady rise in blood sugar levels after eating. The glycemic index is a scale that evaluates carbohydrates according to how quickly they elevate blood sugar levels in comparison to pure glucose, which has a value of 100. Carbohydrate-rich foods with a high GI value (above 70) digest quickly and cause a dramatic increase in blood sugar levels, whereas those with a low GI value (below 55) digest slowly and generate a steady rise in blood sugar levels.

A blood sugar diet typically consists of foods with a lower GI value, which can help manage blood sugar levels and prevent unexpected spikes and falls. This is especially significant for diabetics, as maintaining stable blood sugar levels is critical to their general health and well-being.

Here are some fundamental blood sugar diet principles: Eat low-GI foods, such as whole grains, legumes, non-starchy vegetables, fruits, and lean proteins. These foods digest more slowly, resulting in a more gradual and controlled release of glucose into the bloodstream.

Macronutrient balance: A blood sugar diet focuses on macronutrient balance, specifically carbohydrates, proteins, and fats. A diet that provides an adequate balance of these nutrients aids in the more effective regulation of blood sugar levels.

Portion control: In a blood sugar diet, controlling the portion sizes of meals and snacks is critical. Consuming a lot of carbohydrates, even with a low GI, might cause a spike in blood sugar levels. As a result, controlling portion sizes is critical for maintaining stable blood sugar levels.

Eat regular meals and snacks throughout the day. Eating regular meals and snacks throughout the day can help stabilize blood sugar levels. Meals and snacks should be spaced out every few hours to avoid extended gaps between meals, which can cause blood sugar variations.

Limiting or eliminating sugary and high-GI foods: foods high in added sugars and those with a high GI rating should be limited or eliminated. Examples of these are sugary drinks, candies, pastries, white bread, and sugary cereals, as they can induce a quick rise in blood sugar.

Consider the glycemic load: While the GI is a useful tool, it does not account for food portion sizes. The glycemic load (GL) idea combines the GI value and portion size to provide a more accurate evaluation of a food's impact on blood sugar levels.

Regular physical activity: Physical activity helps to regulate blood sugar levels. Regular physical activity can assist in enhancing insulin sensitivity and glucose uptake by muscles, resulting in better blood sugar control.
It should be noted that a blood sugar diet is particularly suggested for people who have diabetes or are at risk of getting diabetes. It can, however, be advantageous for anyone wanting to maintain stable blood sugar levels and develop good eating habits. To personalize the diet plan and ensure it corresponds with individual needs and goals, check with a healthcare provider or registered dietitian, as with all dietary adjustments.

Benefits of a Blood Sugar Diet

A blood sugar diet, also known as a low-glycemic diet or a diabetic-friendly diet, emphasizes eating foods that do not induce blood sugar rises.

This diet promotes steady blood sugar levels and has several health benefits. Here are some of the advantages of a blood sugar diet:

Blood sugar control: The main advantage of a blood sugar diet is better blood sugar control. Individuals can maintain their glucose levels throughout the day by avoiding foods that rapidly spike blood sugar levels. This is especially important for patients with diabetes or prediabetes because it helps prevent complications caused by uncontrolled blood sugar levels, such as nerve damage, renal difficulties, and cardiovascular disease.

Weight loss and control: A blood sugar diet can help with weight loss and management. Individuals can minimize appetite, feel fuller longer, and avoid overeating by focusing on low-glycemic foods such as whole grains, lean proteins, and veggies. This can result in a calorie deficit and fat loss, assisting individuals in reaching and maintaining a healthy weight.

Enhanced energy levels: Maintaining stable blood sugar levels helps to avoid energy slumps and provides constant energy throughout the day. Low-glycemic-index foods digest more slowly, resulting in a steady release of glucose into the bloodstream. This leads to increased energy and productivity, lowering the need for harmful, high-sugar snacks to battle weariness.

Lessen risk of chronic diseases: When combined with a healthy lifestyle, a blood sugar diet can lessen the chance of acquiring chronic diseases such as type 2 diabetes, heart disease, and some malignancies. Individuals can maintain optimal health and lower their risk of these illnesses by avoiding high-glycemic meals that increase inflammation, insulin resistance, and weight gain.

Better cardiovascular health: A blood sugar diet can improve cardiovascular health by promoting healthy cholesterol levels and lowering the risk of heart disease. High-glycemic meals can cause high cholesterol, high triglycerides, and arterial stiffness. Individuals can maintain good blood lipid profiles and lower their risk of heart disease by eating low-glycemic foods.

Increased brain function: blood sugar levels that are stable also support increased brain function and mental clarity.

Blood sugar changes can cause cognitive impairment, trouble concentrating, and mood swings. Individuals can improve their attention, memory, and overall cognitive performance by eating low-glycemic foods that give a consistent supply of glucose to the brain.

In conclusion, adding low-glycemic items to a blood sugar diet can have a major favorable influence on general health. This type of diet has various advantages, whether for controlling blood sugar levels, obtaining or maintaining a healthy weight, or preventing chronic diseases. Individuals can experience better energy levels, improved cardiovascular health, improved cognitive function, and a lower risk of developing diabetes and other health concerns by making mindful dietary choices.

Getting Started with the Blood Sugar Diet

How to Begin the Blood Sugar Diet

The Blood Sugar Diet is a popular dietary plan that promotes weight loss while regulating blood sugar levels. In order to treat insulin resistance and enhance general health, British physician and author Michael Mosley created this low-calorie, low-carb diet. Whether you want to lose a few pounds or improve your blood sugar control, the Blood Sugar Diet has everything you need to get started.

Understand the Fundamentals: The Blood Sugar Diet is based on a low-calorie, low-carbohydrate diet. It contains components of intermittent fasting, allowing for calorie restriction on certain days. The diet is based on the idea that eating fewer carbohydrates and calories will result in weight loss and better blood sugar control.

Visit your doctor: It is critical to visit your doctor or a certified dietitian before beginning any new diet plan, especially if you have any pre-existing medical conditions or are taking medication.
They can give you specific advice depending on your health situation and needs.

Calculate Your Calorie Intake: Depending on the programme you choose, the Blood Sugar Diet has varied calorie restrictions. The 5:2 Diet and the 800-calorie plan are the most popular options. The 5:2 Diet is eating normally for five days and restricting calorie intake to 500–600 calories on two non-consecutive days. The 800-calorie regimen comprises consuming 800 calories per day for eight weeks. Calculate your calorie requirements and choose the best solution for you.

Select Low-Glycemic Foods: It is critical to consume foods with a low glycemic index (GI) to stabilize blood sugar levels. When compared to high-GI foods, these foods have little effect on blood sugar levels. Include whole grains, legumes, non-starchy veggies, lean proteins, and healthy fats in your diet. Refined carbs, sugary foods, and processed snacks should be avoided.

Practice Intermittent Fasting: An important part of the Blood Sugar Diet is intermittent fasting. It promotes weight loss by activating autophagy, a natural cellular cleaning mechanism. If you're following the 5:2 Diet, choose two non-consecutive days every week to limit your calorie intake. On fasting days, eat low-calorie, nutrient-dense foods like veggies, lean meats, and healthy fats.

Keep an eye on portion sizes: Even while eating low-calorie, low-carb meals, keep an eye on portion proportions. Overeating is easy, especially if you're used to larger servings. Use smaller plates, measure your food, and strive for a balanced dish of vegetables, protein, and healthy fats. It's also important to eat consciously, relishing every bite and paying attention to your body's hunger and satiety signs.

Beware of beverages: The liquids you consume might have a big impact on your blood sugar levels and overall calorie intake. Sugary beverages, such as soda, fruit juices, and sweetened coffee drinks, should be avoided. Instead, drink water, herbal tea, or black coffee. If necessary, limit your alcohol consumption because it contains empty calories and can influence blood sugar stability.

Stay Active: Regular physical activity is a vital component of any healthy lifestyle.
Aerobic exercise, strength training, or any other activity that raises your heart rate can enhance insulin sensitivity,

aid weight loss, and boost overall well-being. Each week, try to get at least 150 minutes of moderate-intensity exercise or 75 minutes of vigorous-intensity activity.

Maintain Consistency: When following the Blood Sugar Diet, consistency is essential. Commit to your chosen calorie restriction programme and stick to it. You will gradually adjust to low-carb, low-calorie meals and reap the benefits of weight loss and blood sugar stabilization. Remember that this is a long-term lifestyle adjustment, not a quick fix.

Seek Support and Resources: Consider joining support groups or online forums where you may get encouragement, tips, and recipe ideas from other Blood Sugar Diet followers. Various books, websites, and apps are also available to help you plan your meals, measure your progress, and learn more about the programme.

Individual outcomes will vary, so consult a healthcare expert before beginning any new diet or exercise programme.
They can provide tailored care based on your individual health needs and objectives.

Chapter 3:
Key Principles of the Blood Sugar Diet

The goal of the low-calorie, low-carb Blood Sugar Diet is to control blood sugar levels in the body to lose weight and enhance general health. Here is a summary of the main ideas of the blood sugar diet:

1. Mediterranean-style, low-carb diet: The Blood Sugar Diet suggests eating a diet rich in fruits, vegetables, whole grains, lean meats, healthy fats, and legumes. The Mediterranean diet is well-liked by those who want to reduce weight, and Dr. Michael Mosley's diet restricts processed carbohydrates and sugary foods while boosting the consumption of whole, nutrient-dense foods. enhance their general health because of its well-established health benefits.

2. Calorie restriction: The diet plan is meant to be modest in calories, with daily caloric intake usually ranging from 800-1,200. By causing a calorie deficit in the body, this calorie restriction aids in the promotion of weight loss. An extremely low-calorie diet may not be appropriate for everyone; therefore, it's crucial to speak with a medical practitioner or qualified dietitian before beginning one.

3. Emphasize low-glycemic index (GI) foods: The Blood Sugar Diet suggests eating foods low in glycemic index (GI) that have little effect on blood sugar levels. Low-GI foods release glucose into the system more gradually because they are absorbed and digested more slowly. Examples of these foods include legumes, whole grains, and non-starchy vegetables. It is simpler to control hunger and cravings when blood sugar levels are stabilized and there are no spikes or crashes.

4. Intermittent fasting: One of the mainstays of the Blood Sugar Diet is intermittent fasting. Eating and fasting are alternated during intermittent fasting. The most popular strategy is called the 5:2 method, in which people eat normally five days a week and limit their calorie intake to 500–600 calories on the other two. This method not only helps with weight loss but may also have positive effects on inflammation and insulin sensitivity.

5. Proper hydration: Maintaining proper hydration is essential for general health and helps control blood sugar levels.
The Blood Sugar Diet suggests drinking a lot of water throughout the day to help the body's metabolic processes and maintain proper hydration levels.

6. Frequent exercise: Getting regular exercise is crucial to following the Blood Sugar Diet. Frequent exercise promotes general cardiovascular health, insulin sensitivity, and calorie burning. To optimize the advantages of the food plan, combine aerobic exercises like brisk walking or biking with strength training.

7. Mindful eating: Eating mindfully entails paying attention to indications of hunger and fullness, eating slowly, and savoring the flavours and textures of food. The Blood Sugar Diet promotes this practice. By reducing overindulgence and emotional eating, mindful eating supports the development of a positive connection with food.

It is crucial to remember that not everyone can follow the Blood Sugar Diet, particularly if they have specific medical issues or dietary restrictions. Before beginning any new diet plan, it is advised to speak with a medical expert or certified dietitian to make sure it is in line with personal health needs and objectives.

Balancing Macronutrients: Carbohydrates, Proteins, and Fats

Maintaining a nutritious diet and reaching general wellness depend heavily on balancing macronutrients, which comprise proteins, lipids, and carbs.

Every macronutrient has a distinct function in the body and offers advantages. The secret to maximizing your nutrition is realizing how important it is to balance these elements.

Our body uses carbohydrates as its main energy source. Upon breakdown, they yield glucose, which powers our brain, muscles, and cells. There are many different types of carbohydrates, including whole grains, fruits, vegetables, and legumes. But not every carbohydrate is made equal. Selecting complex carbs (like quinoa, brown rice, and whole wheat bread) rather than refined carbohydrates (like white bread, candies, and sugary drinks) is crucial. Essential vitamins, minerals, and fiber found in complex carbohydrates aid in blood sugar regulation, digestion, and the promotion of feelings of fullness, which helps curb overeating.

Proteins, the building blocks of our bodies, are essential for tissue growth, healing, and maintenance. They are also essential for many other body processes, including the manufacture of enzymes, the production of hormones, and the operation of the immune system. Lean meats, seafood, eggs, dairy products, legumes, nuts, and seeds are all excellent sources of protein.

A diverse range of protein sources should be incorporated into your diet to guarantee that your body is receiving all the critical amino acids it requires. It's important to balance your protein intake because too much of it might strain your liver and kidneys. Conversely, inadequate protein intake can result in immune system dysfunction, muscular atrophy, and sluggish wound healing.

Although they are sometimes misinterpreted as bad, fats are an essential macronutrient. Fats give us energy, support healthy cell membranes, cushion organs, and aid in the absorption of vitamins. But not every fat is made equally. Essential omega-3 and omega-6 fatty acids are present in healthy fats, which include those found in avocados, nuts, seeds, olive oil, and fatty seafood like salmon and tuna. These fats boost brain function, lower inflammation, and strengthen the heart. Saturated fats, which are present in processed foods and animal products, should be consumed in moderation since they can elevate cholesterol and increase the risk of heart disease. Trans fats, which are harmful to health and are frequently included in packaged and fried foods, should be completely avoided.

To reach a balanced intake of these nutrients, it is recommended to have a well-balanced diet that is diverse and includes all three macronutrients in the appropriate amounts. A balanced plate model can be established by placing fruits and vegetables on half of the plate, items high in protein in the other quarter, and whole grains or complex carbohydrates in the remaining quarter. Achieving a healthy amount of fat in your meals— almonds in salads, for example—or using olive oil as a dressing will help you achieve macronutrient balance.

Recall that dietary requirements could change depending on your age, sex, degree of activity, and general health. To establish a customized plan that fits your unique needs, it is always advisable to speak with a certified dietitian or other healthcare provider. You can provide your body with the energy and nutrition it needs for optimum health and well-being by striking a balance in the amount of macronutrients you consume.

Glycemic Index and Glycemic Load:

Glycemic load (GL) and the glycemic index (GI) are two metrics used to evaluate the effects of various foods on blood sugar levels.

Based on how rapidly they raise blood sugar levels in comparison to pure glucose (which is assigned a value of 100), carbohydrates are ranked in foods according to the Glycemic Index on a scale from 0 to 100. Foods with a high GI digest and absorb quickly, raising blood sugar levels sharply, whereas foods with a low GI absorb and digest more slowly, raising blood sugar levels more gradually and over time.

Conversely, the glycemic load accounts for both the amount and type of carbs in a dish. It is computed by taking the food's GI, multiplying it by the quantity of carbs it contains, and dividing the result by 100. Because this measurement takes into account both the pace of digestion and the actual amount of carbs taken, it offers a more realistic representation of how a certain diet affects blood sugar levels.

For people with diabetes or those trying to control their energy levels, GI and GL are both helpful techniques for controlling blood sugar levels. High-GI and GL foods should be eaten in moderation because they can quickly boost blood sugar levels and then induce an energy crash. On the other hand, foods with low GI and GL absorb and digest more slowly, allowing for a more consistent release of glucose into the bloodstream and stable energy levels.

It is crucial to remember that a variety of factors can affect a food's GI and GL, such as the fruit's level of ripeness, the cooking technique employed, and the inclusion of additional macronutrients (such as fat and protein) that can impede digestion and absorption. As a result, the nutritional values associated with particular foods may not always be precise and may change based on various variables.

A balanced diet rich in a range of low-GI and GL foods, such as fruits, vegetables, whole grains, and legumes, can promote overall health and stable blood sugar levels. However, when considering GI and GL as a guide for meal planning, it is imperative to take into account the individual's unique dietary needs, preferences, and other health issues. Seeking advice from a qualified dietitian or other healthcare expert can offer tailored direction on how to use these measurements efficiently. All things considered, the Glycemic Index and Glycemic Load are useful resources for learning how various foods impact blood sugar levels. People can better control their blood sugar levels and improve their general health by including low- and high-GI items in a balanced diet.

Choosing the Right Foods:

For diabetes management and stable blood sugar levels, selecting the appropriate foods for a blood sugar diet is essential. We may control our blood sugar, lower the risk of problems, and enhance our general health by making educated eating choices.

When choosing foods for a blood sugar diet, keep the following points in mind:

Glycemic Index (GI): This is a system of ratings that indicates how rapidly foods elevate sugar. Eating foods with a low or moderate GI will help you avoid blood sugar spikes. Foods with a high GI should be consumed in moderation or avoided, such as refined carbs and sugary snacks.

Complex Carbohydrates: Whole grains, legumes, and vegetables are good sources of complex carbohydrates because they release glucose into the bloodstream gradually, lowering blood sugar levels. In addition to being high in complex carbs, these fiber-rich foods also help with digestion and satiety.

Lean Proteins: Including lean protein sources in meals, such as beans, fish, poultry, and tofu, will help reduce the rate at which blood sugar is absorbed. Additionally, protein makes you feel fuller for longer, which might help you control your weight.

Healthy Fats: Opt for unsaturated fats from foods like olive oil, avocados, almonds, and seeds. Both cardiovascular health and steady blood sugar levels benefit from these lipids. Steer clear of saturated and trans fats in processed, quick, or fried foods, as they might increase cholesterol and blood sugar.

Portion Control: Although the choice of food is crucial, controlling portion sizes is equally crucial for controlling blood sugar levels. Even eating a lot of healthy foods can make your blood sugar surge. To make sure you are eating the right amounts, pay attention to portion sizes, consult a nutritionist, or use measuring devices.

Regular Meal Timing: People with diabetes need to be consistent about when they eat. Eating throughout the day at regular intervals will help to stabilize blood sugar levels. Strive for three well-balanced meals a day, with healthy snacks as needed, to avoid missing meals.

Customize it: Remember that each individual has a unique body; therefore, meals that suit one person may not suit another. To find out what foods are best for you, try a variety of foods and keep an eye on how your blood sugar responds to them. Seeking advice from a licensed dietician can offer tailored direction and assistance.

In summary, controlling the glycemic load, preserving portion control, and improving nutrition are the key components of selecting the correct foods for a blood sugar diet plan. Incorporating lean proteins, healthy fats, complex carbohydrates, and portion control can help people control their blood sugar levels and enhance their general health.

Portion Control and Meal Timing

Meal timing and portion control are essential elements of a blood sugar diet plan. The goals of this eating strategy are to maintain healthy blood sugar levels, avoid insulin spikes, and enhance general health and well-being.

The concept of portion management describes the habit of eating sensible portions of food at meals and snacks. It entails paying attention to how much food is eaten and making sure that it fits in with one's objectives and nutritional requirements. Portion management teaches people to consume in moderation, preventing overindulgence in calories or overeating.

To properly implement portion control, one must be aware of serving sizes and utilize instruments like food scales, measuring cups, and visual aids. A serving of grains or carbohydrates is roughly the size of a tennis ball, a serving of vegetables is comparable to the size of a baseball, and a suggested quantity of protein is approximately the size of a deck of cards.

Another crucial component of the blood sugar diet plan is the timing of meals. The timing and frequency of meals and snacks have a major impact on blood sugar regulation and weight management. This diet plan often emphasizes eating in a regular, balanced manner throughout the day, with three main meals and two to three short snacks.

By avoiding sharp swings, eating meals at regular intervals contributes to stable blood sugar levels. It also reduces the chance of overeating during meals and guarantees a consistent supply of energy for the body. Furthermore, dividing meals and snacks apart facilitates proper nutrient absorption and digestion.

People following the blood sugar diet are advised to schedule their meals and snacks in advance. This method ensures better portion control and well-balanced meals with lots of protein, healthy fats, and fiber-rich carbohydrates. It is recommended to incorporate a range of foods high in nutrients, including whole grains, nuts, legumes, seafood, and lean meats and vegetables. Additionally, eating meals low in added sugars and high in fiber slows down the body's absorption of glucose, reducing the risk of blood sugar rises. Carbs work best when paired with protein or healthy fats because these macronutrients help stabilize blood sugar and promote satiety.

To sum up, meal planning and portion management are essential components of the blood sugar diet strategy. These routines assist with blood sugar regulation, insulin spike prevention, general health, and weight management. People can better meet their dietary needs and keep stable blood sugar levels throughout the day by eating meals at regular intervals and exercising portion management.

Chapter 4:
Creating a Healthy Meal Plan for Blood Sugar Control

For anyone with diabetes or attempting to control their blood sugar levels, developing a nutritious meal plan is essential. Meals with a variety of nutrients, such as proteins, fats, and carbohydrates, can help stabilize blood sugar levels and reduce the risk of blood sugar spikes. The main ideas of a healthy meal plan for blood sugar control, including food selection, portion sizes, meal scheduling, and possible advantages, will be covered in this extensive guide.

1. Food Selections:

Making the correct dietary choices is essential for controlling blood sugar. Make an effort to include nutrient-dense foods in your diet, such as:

Whole Grains: Because they are higher in fiber and release glucose into the bloodstream more gradually, whole grains like brown rice, quinoa, whole-wheat bread, and oatmeal are the better options.

Lean Proteins: Include low-fat dairy products, fish, chicken, tofu, and lentils in your meals. Proteins aid in reducing the rate at which glucose is absorbed, averting sharp increases in blood sugar levels.

Healthy Fats: Opt for foods like olive oil, avocados, almonds, and seeds that are high in healthy fats. These fats help to balance blood sugar levels, improve insulin sensitivity, and sustain satiety.

Vibrant Vegetables: Include a range of non-starchy veggies in your meals, including carrots, bell peppers, spinach, and broccoli. These veggies are rich in fiber, antioxidants, and other important minerals but low in carbs.

Low-Glycemic Fruits: These fruits, which don't quickly raise blood sugar levels, include berries, apples, oranges, and pears.

2. Measurements of Portion Sizes:

Keep an eye on portion sizes to prevent overindulging, as consuming large amounts of any food can cause blood sugar levels to rise. Appropriate ratios of lipids, proteins, and carbs must be maintained. To make sure you are controlling portions properly, think about using a food scale or measuring cups. You can find out the appropriate portion sizes by speaking with a qualified nutritionist, who will assess your needs and objectives.

3. Timing of Meals:

For blood sugar regulation, a regular eating routine must be established. Try to maintain regular blood sugar levels throughout the day by eating three main meals and two to three healthy snacks at regular intervals. Meal spacing reduces overindulgence and promotes stable energy levels. Meal skipping should be avoided, especially for breakfast, as this might cause blood sugar levels to fluctuate.

4. Meal Structure:

Think about calculating carbs or utilizing the plate technique when organizing your menu. By using the plate technique, you can allocate three-quarters of your plate to lean protein, one-half to non-starchy veggies, and one-quarter to grains or starchy vegetables. This technique regulates portion sizes and guarantees a well-rounded food intake.

Counting carbs entails keeping track of how many are ingested at each meal and adjusting insulin doses accordingly. Effective carbohydrate management helps people regain control over their blood sugar levels.

5. Advantages of a Balanced Diet for Blood Sugar Management:

Following a nutritious diet plan can help control blood sugar in several ways, such as:

Blood Sugar Regulation: A well-balanced diet helps control blood sugar levels, avoiding unexpected rises or falls. People with diabetes or prediabetes need to have this consistency.

Weight Control: Carefully planning meals may help you lose or maintain your weight. Sustaining a healthy weight is crucial for controlling blood sugar levels and lowering the likelihood of acquiring diabetes-related problems.

Heart Health: Nutrient-dense meals low in saturated fats, cholesterol, and sodium are typically included in a healthy meal plan.
This may lessen the chance of cardiovascular illnesses, which are prevalent in diabetics.

Energy Levels: Eating a range of foods high in nutrients guarantees a continuous flow of energy all day long. An appropriately balanced meal plan might help prevent the weariness and lethargic feeling that can result from abrupt blood sugar rises or falls.

General Health: Eating a balanced diet helps regulate blood sugar levels and is good for general health. In addition to strengthening the immune system and lowering the risk of various chronic diseases, a proper diet can also improve digestion and cognitive function. When creating a meal plan for blood sugar control, keep in mind that consulting with a healthcare provider or registered dietitian is essential. They may offer individualized advice based on your unique requirements, health, and way of life. A successful blood sugar management plan also includes lifestyle changes, physical activity, and routine blood sugar monitoring. Adopting a nutritious meal plan can provide substantial benefits for improving blood sugar control and general well-being with dedication and consistency.

Understanding Macronutrient Ratios for Different Goals

The three primary food groups are called macronutrients, or macros for short: fats, proteins, and carbs. Our bodies require certain nutrients to function correctly and stay healthy.

Understanding macronutrient ratios is essential when it comes to the blood sugar diet solution to achieve particular objectives like stabilizing blood sugar levels, decreasing weight, or gaining muscle. You can tailor your diet to get the results you want by adjusting these ratios.

1. Maintaining Healthy Blood Sugar Levels:
The goal of achieving blood sugar stabilization must center on a balanced macronutrient ratio. Generally speaking, a balanced ratio calls for a reasonable intake of proteins, carbs, and healthy fats.

Complex Carbohydrates: These include vegetables high in fiber, lentils, and whole grains. Because these carbohydrates break down more slowly, blood sugar spikes are avoided.

Proteins: Choose lean protein sources such as tofu, fish, eggs, and poultry. Proteins support long-lasting energy and blood sugar regulation.

Fats: Include unsaturated fats from foods like olive oil, avocados, nuts, and seeds. By slowing down digestion, these fats help to avoid sharp rises in blood sugar.

2. Loss of weight:

Macronutrient ratios are crucial for establishing a calorie deficit and preserving vital nutrients when trying to lose weight.

Cut Down on Carbs: Cutting back on carbohydrates may force the body to burn fat that has been stored as energy. Reduce your intake of refined sugars and increase your intake of complex carbs.

Eat More Protein: Since protein increases feelings of fullness and helps to build lean muscle mass, it is essential for weight loss. Pick lean protein sources, including fish, poultry, low-fat dairy, and plant-based foods like quinoa and lentils.

Add healthy fats: Including healthy fats is crucial for promoting hormonal balance and fullness. Think about things like almonds, seeds, avocados, and fatty fish like salmon.

3. Building Muscle:

A blood sugar diet solution makes it possible to gain muscle mass, but it also makes it necessary to modify the macronutrient ratios to supply enough energy and nutrients for muscle growth.

Up Your Protein Intake: Building and repairing muscles need protein. Lean meats, dairy products, lentils, and plant-based protein sources can all help you consume more protein.

Moderate Carbohydrates: Carbs help burn fat during exercise and refuel your muscles' glycogen stores. When it comes to maintaining energy levels during vigorous workouts, concentrate on complex carbs found in whole grains, fruits, and starchy vegetables.

Healthy Fats: Add healthy fats to your diet because they help produce hormones and provide you with the energy you need. It is advised to use foods like avocados, almonds, and olive oil.

Keep in mind that your unique goals, preferences, and any underlying medical concerns should all be taken into account when determining your macronutrient ratios. You can find the best macronutrient ratios for you and be guided toward a healthy blood sugar diet solution by speaking with a qualified dietitian or nutritionist.

Building Balanced Meals and Snacks

Building balanced meals and snacks is vital for maintaining stable blood sugar levels, especially for those following a blood sugar diet solution. The major purpose of this diet is to keep blood sugar levels within a healthy range by eliminating high glycemic foods and including a variety of nutrient-dense options.

When preparing a meal or snack, it is vital to incorporate a balance of macronutrients such as carbohydrates, proteins, and healthy fats. This helps slow down the digestion and absorption of carbs, minimizing rapid rises in blood sugar levels.

Carbohydrates are a main source of energy, but not all carbs are equal. Foods with a low glycemic index (GI) are recommended as they promote a slower rise in blood glucose levels. Examples of low GI carbs include whole grains like oats, quinoa, and brown rice, as well as non-starchy vegetables like leafy greens, broccoli, and cauliflower. These should form the cornerstone of your meals.

Protein has a critical role in maintaining blood sugar stability as it helps slow down the absorption of carbs. Include lean sources of protein, such as chicken, turkey, fish, tofu, lentils, and eggs. These can be mixed with the low GI carbs to produce a balanced meal.

Healthy fats, such as avocados, nuts, seeds, and olive oil, are beneficial for producing satiety and decreasing the overall glycemic load of a meal or snack. Including a small portion of healthy fats in your meals will help balance blood sugar levels and provide long-lasting energy.

In addition to macronutrients, including fiber-rich foods in your meals and snacks is advantageous. Fiber helps slow down the digestion and absorption of carbs, reducing fast blood sugar increases. Incorporate fiber-rich fruits like berries, apples, and oranges, as well as vegetables, nuts, and seeds.

When it comes to snacking, preparing ahead is crucial. Opt for whole food selections rather than packaged snacks heavy in sugar and bad fats. Some examples of balanced snacks for blood sugar regulation may be a handful of almonds with a piece of fruit, celery sticks with almond butter or hummus, a small bit of Greek yogurt with berries, or a cooked egg with raw veggies.

Remember to also watch portion quantities and eat thoughtfully. It's crucial to listen to your body's hunger and fullness signs and prevent overeating. Eating modest, regular meals and snacks throughout the day can also help maintain stable blood sugar levels.

In conclusion, establishing balanced meals and snacks for a blood sugar diet solution requires integrating low-GI carbohydrates, lean proteins, healthy fats, and fiber-rich foods.

By focusing on nutrient-dense selections and avoiding processed foods, you may efficiently manage your blood sugar levels and enhance your overall health and well-being.

Meal Prepping and Grocery Shopping Tips

Meal Preparation and Grocery Shopping Tips for Blood Sugar Diet Solution

Maintaining normal blood sugar levels is vital for our general health and well-being. By choosing a blood sugar diet plan, we can efficiently manage our blood sugar levels and achieve maximum health. Here are some meal preparation and grocery shopping recommendations to aid you in your quest for a healthier blood sugar diet solution.

Plan Ahead: Before heading to the grocery store, spend some time planning your meals for the week. This can help you construct a shopping list of the necessary ingredients and prevent impulse purchases of bad meals. Designate certain days for different meals and take into account your dietary requirements and preferences.

Fill Your Cart with Whole Foods: When shopping, focus on whole foods that are naturally low in sugar and have a low glycemic index. Choose lean proteins such as chicken, turkey, fish, and tofu. Opt for complex carbs like brown rice, quinoa, and whole-grain bread. Fill your cart with fiber-rich veggies like spinach, broccoli, and kale, and don't forget to include a variety of fresh fruits.

Examine labels thoroughly: Take the time to thoroughly examine the food labels of the things you buy. Check for hidden sugars, artificial sweeteners, or unhealthy ingredients. Avoid processed foods that generally contain excessive amounts of added sugars and harmful fats.

Choose Healthy Fats: Incorporate healthy fats into your diet, such as avocados, nuts, seeds, and olive oil. These fats can help slow down the absorption of sugar into your system, keeping your blood sugar levels constant.

Shop the perimeter: The outside aisles of the grocery store are often where you'll find fresh vegetables, lean proteins, and dairy goods. Spend most of your time in these regions, as they offer nutrient-rich foods that are vital for maintaining stable blood sugar levels.

Control Portion Sizes: To manage blood sugar levels successfully, it's vital to watch your portion sizes. Prepare your meals with suitable serving sizes, and utilize containers or meal prep storage to portion out your meals for easy access during the week. This will help you avoid overeating and make healthier choices.

Cook at home: By making your meals at home, you have full control over what goes into your dishes. Avoid dining out as much as possible, as restaurant meals often contain hidden sweets and harmful components that can induce blood sugar spikes.

Use Flavorful Spices: Instead of relying on artificial sauces and condiments, try using natural herbs and spices to add flavor to your meals. Cinnamon can help manage blood sugar levels, while turmeric has anti-inflammatory qualities. Get inventive with varied flavors to make your meals fascinating and enjoyable.

Bulk Cooking: Save time and ensure you have healthy options available by bulk cooking. Prepare greater quantities of meals that may be refrigerated and reheated throughout the week. This will keep you from succumbing to unhealthy fast-food selections during hectic days.

Stay Hydrated: Hydration plays a critical part in controlling blood sugar levels. Drink enough water throughout the day to maintain your body's functioning and aid with digestion. Limit your intake of sugary beverages and go for herbal teas or infused water instead.

By applying these meal preparation and grocery shopping methods, you can take control of your blood sugar diet solution. With careful planning, smart buying, and tasty cooked meals, you'll be on your way to maintaining stable blood sugar levels and promoting a healthier lifestyle.

Chapter 5:
Blood Sugar-Friendly Recipes and Meal Ideas

Maintaining healthy blood sugar levels is vital for managing diabetes or preventing its occurrence. Creating meals that are low in sugar and carbohydrates and rich in fiber and protein will help regulate blood sugar levels. Here are some blood sugar-friendly dishes and meal ideas to integrate into your diet:

1. Breakfast:

Veggie omelet: Use egg whites or a combination of whole eggs and egg whites, and incorporate plenty of low-carb vegetables, including spinach, peppers, mushrooms, and onions.

Greek yogurt with berries: Choose plain Greek yogurt and top it with fresh berries, which are low in sugar, antioxidants, and fiber.

2. Lunch:

Grilled chicken salad: Start with a bed of leafy greens; add grilled chicken breast, cherry tomatoes, cucumbers, and avocado. Dress with a homemade vinaigrette using vinegar, olive oil, and herbs.

Lentil soup: Incorporate high-fiber lentils into a vegetable soup with carrots, celery, onions, garlic, and low-sodium broth.

3. Snacks: Almonds and walnuts, These nuts provide healthy fats, protein, and fiber, which help manage blood sugar levels. Enjoy a handful as a filling snack.
Veggie sticks with hummus, carrots, celery, cucumbers, and bell peppers dipped in hummus create a healthy and enjoyable snack.

4. Dinner: Baked salmon, Season wild-caught salmon with herbs and spices, then bake or broil it. Serve with a side of roasted Brussels sprouts and quinoa.
Stir-fried tofu and veggies: Choose nutrient-rich vegetables such as broccoli, bell peppers, snap peas, and mushrooms, then stir-fry them with tofu in a low-sodium soy sauce.

5. Dessert: Sugar-free chia pudding, Mix chia seeds with unsweetened almond milk, a sugar alternative, and vanilla extract. Refrigerate overnight and eat, topped with berries.
Baked apple with cinnamon: core an apple, sprinkle with cinnamon and a splash of stevia and bake until soft.
Serve warm with a dollop of Greek yogurt.
Remember to focus on portion control and choose whole, unprocessed foods. These recipes and meal ideas

can be adapted to individual preferences or dietary constraints, ensuring they are blood sugar-friendly and enjoyable for everyone.

Breakfast Recipes for Stable Blood Sugar

If you or someone you love struggles with fluctuating blood sugar levels, it's crucial to choose breakfast recipes that are low in added sugars and high in complex carbohydrates, fiber, and protein. These recipes will help ensure a consistent release of glucose into the system, preventing spikes and decreases in blood sugar levels. Here are some great breakfast recipes to help balance blood sugar:

1. Quinoa Breakfast Bowl:

- Ingredients:

1/2 cup cooked quinoa

1/4 cup unsweetened almond milk

1 tablespoon chopped nuts (such as almonds or walnuts)

1 tablespoon unsweetened coconut flakes; 1/4 cup mixed berries

- Instructions:

1. In a bowl, mix the cooked quinoa and almond milk.

2. Top with chopped nuts, coconut flakes, and mixed berries.

3. Stir gently to mix.

4. Serve at room temperature or cooled.

2. Greek Yogurt and Berry Parfait:
- Ingredients:
1 cup Greek yogurt (unsweetened)
1/4 cup mixed berries (blueberries, raspberries, strawberries)
1 tablespoon chopped nuts (almonds, walnuts)
1 tablespoon chia seeds

- Instructions:
1. In a small glass or bowl, layer the Greek yogurt, mixed berries, almonds, and chia seeds.
2. Repeat the layers until all ingredients are utilized.
3. Serve cold.

3. Veggie and Egg Scramble:
- Ingredients:
2 eggs
1/4 cup sliced bell peppers (mixed colors)
1/4 cup chopped onions
1/4 cup chopped mushrooms
1 tablespoon olive oil
Salt and pepper to taste

- Instructions:
1. In a small bowl, whisk the eggs until fully beaten.
2. Heat the olive oil in a non-stick skillet over medium heat.

3. Add the onions, bell peppers, and mushrooms. Sauté until softened.

4. Pour the beaten eggs over the vegetables in the skillet. Season with salt and pepper.

5. Cook the scramble until the eggs are set, stirring periodically.

4. Avocado and Whole Grain Toast:
- Ingredients:
1 slice whole grain bread (toasted)
1/2 ripe avocado
1 boiled egg, sliced
Salt and pepper to taste

- Instructions:
1. Spread the ripe avocado equally over the toasted bread piece.

2. Season with salt and pepper.

3. Arrange the sliced, boiled egg on top of the avocado.

4. Sprinkle with additional salt and pepper, if required.

5. Green Smoothie with Spinach and Protein:
- Ingredients:
1 cup spinach leaves
1/2 cup unsweetened almond milk
1/2 frozen banana
1 tablespoon almond butter
1 scoop vanilla protein powder (low sugar)

1/2 cup ice cubes

- Instructions:

1. In a blender, combine the spinach, almond milk, frozen banana, almond butter, protein powder, and ice cubes.

2. Blend until smooth and creamy.

3. Pour into a glass and enjoy immediately.

Remember to alter these recipes according to your nutritional needs, or visit a healthcare expert or certified dietitian if you have special concerns about your blood sugar levels. Maintaining stable blood sugar is vital for overall health, and a healthy breakfast can play a big part in accomplishing this aim.

Lunch and Dinner Recipes for Balanced Blood Sugar

For people with diabetes or insulin resistance in particular, maintaining regulated blood sugar levels is critical to general health. Meal plans that have a balance of fiber, healthy fats, lean protein, and complex carbohydrates will help control blood sugar levels and give you energy all day. The following dishes for lunch and dinner can help to maintain balanced blood sugar levels:

1. Salad with Grilled Chicken:

3–4 ounces of grilled chicken breast

Mixed greens

Cherry tomatoes

Slices of cucumber

Avocado slices

A dressing made of Greek yogurt, lemon juice, olive oil, garlic, salt, and pepper.

2. Quinoa with Roasted Vegetables and Baked Salmon:

A fresh filet of salmon

Lemon juice

Powdered garlic

Pepper and salt

Half a cup of quinoa

A variety of veggies, such as bell peppers, broccoli, zucchini, etc.

Olive oil

Fresh herbs (basil, thyme, and rosemary)

3. Stir-fried Turkey with Veggies:

Turkey ground (4-6 oz)

Olive oil

Onion

Cloves of garlic

A variety of vegetables, such as carrots, cauliflower, snap peas, and bell peppers

Soy sauce with low sodium

Sesame oil
Powdered ginger
Almond slices, if desired

4. Soup with Lentils and Vegetables:
One cup of dried lentils
Onion
Cloves of garlic
Carrots
Celery
Kale or spinach
Reduced-sodium vegetable stock
Olive oil;
Dried herbs (bay leaves, thyme, and rosemary)
Pepper and salt

5. Stuffed Bell Peppers with Quinoa:
Bell peppers (mixture of hues)
Half a cup of quinoa
3–4 ounces of ground lean chicken or turkey
Onion
Cloves of garlic
Low-sugar tomato sauce
Fresh herbs, such as basil and parsley
Pepper and salt

Optional: shredded mozzarella cheese

Keep an eye on portion sizes and make adjustments to your specific dietary requirements. To support the best possible blood sugar control, it's also critical to combine these meals with frequent exercise, hydration, and a balanced lifestyle. For individualized guidance, speak with a qualified dietitian or other medical practitioner.

Snacks and Desserts that won't Spike Blood Sugar

Maintaining stable blood sugar levels is critical for people with diabetes or those looking to regulate their overall sugar intake. Here are some appetizers and sweets that won't produce a big surge in blood sugar levels:

1. Fresh fruit: Enjoy a range of naturally sweet fruits, including berries, apples, pears, or citrus fruits. These fruits include fiber that slows down sugar absorption, avoiding blood sugar rises.

2. Nuts and seeds: Nuts and seeds, such as almonds, walnuts, chia seeds, or flaxseeds, are rich with healthy fats, cholesterol, and fiber. This combination helps slow down the flow of sugar into the bloodstream.

3. Greek yogurt: A cup of unsweetened Greek yogurt gives a sufficient quantity of protein without excessive sugar. You can top it with sliced fruit or a sprinkling of cinnamon for added taste.

4. Sugar-free or dark chocolate: Opt for sugar-free or dark chocolate with at least 70% cocoa. Dark chocolate is lower in sugar and has more fiber, making it a better choice for maintaining stable blood sugar.

5. Veggie sticks with hummus: Combine fiber-rich veggies like carrot sticks, cucumber slices, or bell pepper strips with a small serving of hummus. It provides a tasty snack without dramatically influencing blood sugar levels.

6. Sugar-free gelatin or pudding: These sweets are manufactured with sugar replacements and can be a guilt-free pleasure for individuals watching their blood sugar levels. Just make sure to choose the sugar-free options and consume them in moderation.

7. Homemade trail mix: Create a unique trail mix with unsalted nuts, seeds, and a large amount of dried fruit. This combination provides a balance of protein, healthy fats, and natural carbohydrates while keeping blood sugar under check.

8. Rice cakes with nut butter: Whole grain rice cakes provide a low glycemic index alternative, meaning they won't produce a sudden surge in blood sugar levels. Add a thin layer of nut butter for extra taste and healthy fats.

9. Popcorn: Opt for air-popped popcorn or mildly seasoned types with no extra sugar. Popcorn is a whole-grain snack that can deliver a pleasing crunch and fiber without triggering major blood sugar swings.

10. Chia pudding: Chia seeds can absorb liquid and produce a gel-like consistency, making them great for creating a pudding or a creamy dessert. Mix them with unsweetened almond milk, vanilla extract, and a natural low-calorie sweetener for a tasty and blood sugar-friendly treat.

Remember, portion control is necessary even while consuming snacks and desserts with moderate sugar impacts. Paying attention to the overall carbohydrate content of foods and spreading them equally throughout the day can also aid in maintaining blood sugar levels successfully.

Chapter 6:
Incorporating Exercise and Physical Activity

A healthy lifestyle requires us to include physical activity and exercise in our everyday routines. Exercise not only increases our physical fitness but also has many positive effects on our general wellbeing and mental health. The following are some practical strategies for integrating physical activity and fitness into our daily lives:

1. Choose enjoyable activities: Finding enjoyable hobbies is essential to maintaining a fitness regimen. There are several activities available, including running, cycling, swimming, dancing, playing sports, and yoga. Fitting exercise into your everyday schedule will be made easier if you find enjoyable and interesting hobbies.

It's also critical to pay attention to your body and take days off when necessary. Burnout and injury can result from pushing yourself too hard or overexerting yourself. When exercising, be aware of any pain or discomfort and adjust or get professional help if needed.

It's not only about regimented workouts—you can include physical activity and exercise into your everyday life. It can also entail making little lifestyle adjustments, like choosing to walk during your lunch break, use the stairs instead of the elevator, or go for a bike ride instead of driving. Over time, these minor modifications might accumulate and enhance your overall level of fitness.

There are several advantages to regular exercise for your bodily and emotional well-being. It strengthens muscles, increases cardiovascular health, and improves endurance and flexibility. Known as "feel-good" hormones, endorphins are also released during exercise and can help lower stress, anxiety, and depressive symptoms.

Regular exercise can also increase energy, improve the quality of sleep, and improve cognitive function. It can boost self-confidence and general happiness in addition to improving focus and productivity. Including physical activity and exercise in your routine can also help you control your weight and lower your chance of developing chronic illnesses including heart disease, type 2 diabetes, and some cancers.

In summary, it is essential to include physical activity and exercise in your daily routine in order to maintain a healthy lifestyle. Integrating exercise into your life successfully requires finding fun activities, establishing reasonable goals, prioritizing fitness, and exercising flexibility. Making your overall health a priority will allow you to reap the many advantages that come with engaging in regular physical activity.

2. Make reasonable goals for yourself: Begin small and make reasonable goals for yourself. As you gain strength and endurance, gradually increase the length and intensity of your workouts. Always keep in mind that small amounts of activity throughout the day can have a significant impact.

3. Give it top priority: Include exercise in your daily schedule without exception. Make it a priority by setting aside time for exercise. Choose a time that works best for you and stick with it, whether it's in the morning, during lunch breaks, or at night.

4. Make physical activity a part of your everyday tasks: Seek for chances to move your body throughout the day. Use the stairs rather than the elevator. If you can, try to bike or walk to work. When you're done working at your desk, take brief walks or pauses to stretch. Your total level of fitness can be significantly affected by these tiny adjustments.

5. Find a workout partner: Exercising with a partner can boost motivation and increase enjoyment. Find a family member or acquaintance who is as motivated by fitness as you are, and plan frequent training sessions with them. You can encourage one another to stick to your fitness regimen and turn it into a group activity.

6. Mix it up: Vary your workout regimen to stay interesting and maintain motivation. Take advantage of group fitness courses, experiment with different regimens, and discover new environments. This diversity will keep things fresh and focus on various muscle groups for a more well-rounded exercise program.

7. Make use of technology: Make use of wearables or fitness applications to measure your heart rate, steps, and calories burned while exercising, as well as to set objectives and track your progress. These resources can be used as motivational tools and as a source of insightful criticism.

8. Be adaptive and flexible: Maintaining a regular workout schedule might be difficult when life gets busy. Be adaptable throughout these periods and come up with other ways to get exercise into your day. It might be as easy as walking briefly, doing bodyweight exercises at home, or watching an internet fitness video.
Always remember that finding what works best for you and being consistent are the keys to incorporating exercise and physical activity. Including exercise in your daily regimen will help you achieve better overall health, mental clarity, and physical fitness.

The Role of Exercise in Blood Sugar Regulation

Exercise on a regular basis is essential for controlling blood sugar, particularly in those who have diabetes or pre-diabetes. Engaging in physical activity not only enhances blood sugar regulation but also lowers the risk of diabetic complications and enhances general health.

The capacity of exercise to improve insulin sensitivity is one of the main advantages for blood sugar regulation. The hormone insulin is in charge of controlling blood sugar levels by permitting glucose to enter cells. However, the body's cells become less sensitive to insulin in those who have diabetes or insulin resistance. Regular exercise stimulates the muscles, making them more capable of utilizing glucose without the need for insulin. Better glycemic management and decreased blood sugar levels may result from this enhanced insulin sensitivity.

Exercise can also aid in weight management, which is another important factor in controlling blood sugar. Being overweight, particularly in the belly, is linked to insulin resistance and a higher chance of type 2 diabetes. Engaging in regular physical activity lowers the risk of diabetes and improves blood sugar control by burning calories, encouraging fat reduction, and maintaining a healthy weight.

The energy that the muscles need for exercise comes from glucose that is stored in the muscles and liver. Consequently, exercise helps the body eliminate extra glucose from the blood, which lowers blood sugar levels. Furthermore, muscle glycogen synthesis and availability are both enhanced by exercise. When needed, glucose can be swiftly transformed from glycogen, a form of glucose that has been stored. This enhanced ability to store glycogen may help the body react better to elevated blood sugar levels.

The ability of exercise to lower insulin demand in people with type 1 diabetes is another advantage for blood sugar regulation. Frequent exercise can improve insulin absorption, increasing the insulin's effectiveness when given. Better glucose control and a lower risk of problems associated with insulin use can be attained by those with type 1 diabetes by doing this.

Exercise also provides a host of cardiovascular advantages, all of which are critical for people with diabetes. It is well recognized that diabetes raises the risk of stroke and heart disease. Frequent exercise lowers blood pressure, raises circulation, lowers cholesterol, and strengthens the heart, all of which assist to lessen the risk of cardiovascular problems.

Selecting pleasurable and long-lasting activities is crucial to maximizing the advantages of exercise on blood sugar management. A comprehensive strategy to blood sugar control can involve combining strength training activities with cardiovascular activities like biking, swimming, running, or walking. To guarantee safe and efficient glucose control, blood sugar levels must be monitored before, during, and following exercise, particularly for those using diabetes medication.

In summary, blood sugar management in those with diabetes or pre-diabetes is greatly aided by exercise. It enhances insulin sensitivity, helps control weight, expels extra glucose from the blood, lowers insulin needs, and has positive effects on the cardiovascular system. Frequent exercise can greatly improve blood sugar control, lower the risk of problems, and improve general health and well-being when paired with adequate medical therapy.

Types of Exercises for Blood Sugar Control

For those with diabetes, exercise is a good strategy to control blood sugar levels. Frequent exercise improves insulin sensitivity, decreases blood sugar, increases the body's ability to use insulin, and lowers the chance of developing problems related to diabetes. The following workout regimens are helpful for controlling blood sugar:

Aerobic workouts: By raising heart rate and burning calories, these exercises help people maintain a healthy weight and enhance cardiovascular health. Walking quickly, running, swimming, cycling, dancing, and aerobic classes are a few examples. Try to get in at least 150 minutes a week, spread out over three days, of moderate-intensity aerobic exercise.

Resistance training: Exercises that build muscle mass and improve insulin sensitivity help to better regulate blood sugar. These workouts consist of bodyweight movements like lunges, squats, and push-ups as well as the use of weights and resistance bands. Aim for two to three strength training sessions per week, focusing on the main muscle groups.

High-intensity interval training (HIIT): HIIT consists of brief bursts of vigorous activity interspersed with rest intervals. Compared to conventional, constant-paced exercises, this kind of exercise has been demonstrated to increase insulin sensitivity and reduce blood sugar levels more successfully. Running, riding, and using exercise devices like rowing machines or treadmills are a few examples. However, because of the possible hazards, people with diabetes should speak with their healthcare provider before beginning HIIT.

Yoga: Yoga incorporates meditation, breathing techniques, and physical postures. It can ease tension, increase suppleness, and encourage unwinding. Some yoga poses, like twists, forward bends, and standing poses, may help regulate blood sugar levels. In addition to improving general health, yoga can help control blood sugar swings brought on by stress.

Water exercises: These types of workouts are easy on the joints and offer a low-impact workout. Strengthening, stretching, and increasing cardiovascular fitness can all be achieved through swimming, water aerobics, and walking. Those with restricted mobility or joint issues can participate in these activities.

Sports: Playing sports, whether on a team or an individual basis, can be a fun approach to get more exercise. Sports including tennis, golf, basketball, soccer, volleyball, and soccer assist lower blood sugar levels while enhancing cardiovascular health, strength, and coordination.

It is crucial to remember that before beginning an exercise program, people with diabetes should speak with their healthcare physician or a diabetes educator. They can offer tailored advice depending on a person's exercise level, blood sugar control objectives, and current state of health. In order to avoid hypoglycemia, it is also crucial to check blood sugar levels prior to, during, and following exercise (low blood sugar). Doses of insulin or medications may need to be changed accordingly.

In conclusion, people with diabetes can benefit from a variety of exercise regimens that assist regulate their blood sugar levels.

A regular exercise program can improve insulin sensitivity, lower blood sugar, and improve general well-being by combining aerobic workouts, resistance training, HIIT, yoga, water exercises, and sports activities. To make sure a new fitness program is safe and appropriate for their needs, people should speak with their healthcare physician before beginning. To avoid hypoglycemia during exercise, it's also critical to monitor blood sugar levels and alter medicine or insulin dosage as needed.

To maintain ideal blood sugar control, the crucial thing is to identify pleasurable activities that you can engage in on a regular basis. Always start out cautiously, build up the duration and intensity of your workouts gradually, and pay attention to your body. Frequent exercise can significantly help control blood sugar levels and lower the risk of complications from diabetes when paired with a nutritious diet and other lifestyle changes.

Developing an Exercise Routine for Long-term Success

Creating an Exercise Program for Diabetes Patients to Achieve Long-Term Success

Getting regular exercise is crucial for controlling diabetes and enhancing general health. Exercise improves heart health, helps people manage their weight, lowers stress, and increases energy in those with diabetes. It also helps control blood sugar levels. However, it takes deliberate thought and preparation to design a fitness program that helps diabetics succeed over the long run. The following are some essential elements to take into account while creating an exercise program for long-term success:

Speak with a healthcare provider: It is essential to speak with a healthcare provider—ideally an exercise physiologist or a diabetic specialist—before beginning any kind of fitness regimen. They can assess your condition, identify any restrictions, and provide recommendations tailored to your unique requirements and objectives. They can also offer pertinent advice and assist you in identifying any possible concerns related to exercise.

Select a range of workouts: Including a range of workouts in your regimen guarantees that various muscle groups are used and helps you avoid becoming bored. Aerobic workouts like brisk walking, cycling, swimming, or dancing should be a part of a balanced program to improve insulin sensitivity and cardiovascular health. Incorporating resistance band or weight machine workouts into your strength training regimen can help you gain muscle growth, maintain joint health, and improve your metabolism overall.

Establish attainable goals: Maintaining long-term success requires setting realistic goals. To begin, choose modest, quantifiable goals that correspond with your overall health objectives. For example, try to do 30 minutes of aerobic activity at a moderate level at least five days a week. Increase the length or intensity of your workouts progressively as you advance. Always keep in mind that even little workouts spread throughout the day can help with better blood sugar control.

Check blood sugar levels: In order to make sure their levels stay within a healthy range, people with diabetes must be sure to check their blood sugar levels before, during, and after activity. Monitoring enables you to see how your body reacts to various activities and makes necessary modifications to medication, diet schedules, and exercise intensity. Maintaining a record of your workouts and blood sugar levels can give you important information that will support your decision-making.

Remain hydrated: Adequate hydration is important for everyone, but it's especially important for diabetics when they exercise. Maintaining adequate hydration promotes healthy blood volume and circulation, controls body temperature, and supports efficient metabolic processes. Try to stay hydrated before, during, and after your workouts. For individualized recommendations on hydration, speak with your healthcare provider if you have any other medical issues or are taking any medications that may impact your fluid balance. Think about scheduling and keeping an eye on your symptoms: When you exercise, the time of day might affect how your body reacts to physical activity. To create a routine, try to arrange your workouts for the same time every day. Keeping an eye on how your body reacts when exercising is equally crucial. Watch out for symptoms like weakness, dizziness, excessive perspiration, or strange changes in eyesight as these could mean that you should modify the amount of time or intensity that you exercise. Inform your healthcare provider right once if you experience any odd symptoms.

Include rest days: Your body needs time to recuperate from and adjust to the physical strain of exercise. Include rest days in your schedule to allow your muscles to regenerate. On rest days, doing simple exercises like yoga or stretching can help you stay flexible and avoid being tight.

Regularly review and modify: As your fitness journey advances, review and modify your workout regimen on a regular basis to keep pushing yourself and stay away from plateaus. Periodically increase the length or intensity of your workouts to ensure that your body is always adapting. Furthermore, review your objectives to make sure they still meet your evolving health needs and are relevant, attainable, and in line with your aspirations. Personalized planning and ongoing supervision are essential for developing a fitness program that will work for diabetes in the long run. By adhering to these recommendations, seeking advice from medical specialists, and maintaining consistency, you may create a routine that promotes ideal blood sugar control, enhances general health, and guarantees long-term sustainability.

Chapter 7:
Managing Stress and Sleep for Healthy Blood Sugar Levels

Keeping blood sugar levels in a healthy range requires both stress management and adequate sleep. Your body's capacity to control blood sugar can be severely compromised by high stress levels and sleep deprivation, which increases your risk of developing diabetes and insulin resistance. The following advice will help you better sleep and manage stress in order to support normal blood sugar levels:

1. Stress reduction methods:
- Engage in relaxation exercises like yoga, meditation, and deep breathing. Blood sugar levels can rise when stress chemicals like cortisol are released, but these exercises can help lower them.
- Exercise on a regular basis; it's a natural way to reduce stress. Include an enjoyable hobby in your daily routine.
- Throughout the day, take breaks to engage in activities you enjoy, such as reading, listening to music, or spending time with close friends and family. Taking part in enjoyable activities can assist in lowering stress levels.

2. Make sleep a priority:

- Even on weekends, stick to a regular sleep schedule by going to bed and waking up at the same time every day. This enhances the quality of your sleep by assisting in the regulation of your body's internal clock.

- Make sure your bedroom is calm, cold, and dark to promote good sleep. Purchase cozy cushions and bedding, and keep all distracting objects like bright lights and electronics out of the room. Steer clear of stimulants and coffee in the evening since they may impede your ability to fall asleep. Before going to bed, consider using relaxing methods or herbal drinks like chamomile.

- Minimize the amount of time spent on laptops or smartphones right before bed. These devices' blue light emissions can interfere with your body's normal circadian rhythm and make it more difficult to fall asleep.

3. Nutritious eating practices:

- Include a diet high in fruits, vegetables, whole grains, lean proteins, and balance. This will assist in regulating blood sugar levels all day long.

- Steer clear of missing meals since this may cause blood sugar levels to fluctuate. Consume well-balanced meals on a regular basis, along with wholesome snacks, to avoid energy dips and sugar cravings.

- Restrict your intake of sugary drinks, processed foods, and sugary snacks. These can have a detrimental effect on your overall blood sugar control by causing quick rises in blood sugar levels that are followed by crashes.
- Drink lots of water throughout the day to stay hydrated. Dehydration can lead to feelings of exhaustion and tension as well as have an impact on blood sugar management.

Your body can regulate blood sugar levels far better if you control your stress levels and make sleep a priority. Make these suggestions part of your everyday routine to live a more balanced and healthful life. For tailored counsel and direction, it's crucial to speak with a healthcare expert.
It's also important to remember that you should always seek the counsel and direction of a healthcare provider if you have any current medical conditions or concerns about your blood sugar levels. Based on your unique situation, they can provide you with the most suitable and accurate recommendations.

The Impact of Stress on Blood Sugar

People of all ages and backgrounds experience stress, which seems to be an inherent aspect of modern life. Numerous things might cause it, including pressures from the workplace, interpersonal connections, financial hardships, and health problems. Excessive or chronic stress can negatively impact our general health, including blood sugar disturbance, even though stress is a natural reaction meant to protect and inspire us.

The pancreas secretes the hormone insulin, which is crucial for regulating blood sugar levels. Insulin assists in transferring blood glucose into cells so that it can be utilized as an energy source. Stress, however, causes physiological and hormonal alterations that can impair insulin's efficiency and cause an imbalance in blood sugar levels.

Stress hormones like cortisol and adrenaline are released by the body when it experiences stress, which triggers the fight-or-flight reaction. These hormones cause the liver to manufacture and release glucose into the bloodstream, which raises blood sugar levels. This process is meant to give the body an energy boost when faced with difficult circumstances.

Chronic stress, however, can cause cortisol levels to rise for an extended period of time, which can disrupt insulin's regular activity. Cortisol has the ability to decrease insulin's ability to move glucose from the bloodstream into cells by strengthening cell resistance to its actions. Blood sugar levels may therefore continue to rise, which may eventually cause prediabetes or type 2 diabetes.

Furthermore, emotional eating and unhealthy coping strategies are two more ways that stress can have an indirect effect on blood sugar. High-calorie comfort foods are a common choice for people who are stressed, and they can quickly raise blood sugar levels. This is referred to as "stress eating," and it frequently entails consuming fatty or sugary meals that may temporarily alleviate symptoms but may also lead to chronic blood sugar abnormalities.

In addition, stress can affect hunger, sleep patterns, and physical activity levels—all of which can have an impact on blood sugar regulation. Insufficient sleep has been associated with heightened inflammation and insulin resistance, impeding the body's ability to effectively metabolize glucose.

Sustaining ideal blood sugar levels requires effective stress management. The negative effects of stress on the body can be lessened by implementing stress-reduction strategies including deep breathing exercises, frequent exercise, meditation, or taking up a hobby. Furthermore, reducing stress and promoting general well-being can be greatly aided by forming support networks, getting expert assistance, and engaging in self-care.

In summary, blood sugar levels are impacted by stress both directly and indirectly. The efficacy of insulin may be compromised by prolonged or severe stress, which can result in abnormalities in the management of blood sugar. Furthermore, stress-related behaviors such as emotional eating, inactivity, and restless nights can also lead to variations in blood sugar levels. Maintaining ideal blood sugar levels and general health requires acknowledging and properly handling stress.

Stress-Management Techniques for Stable Blood Sugar

Blood sugar levels can be greatly impacted by stress, particularly in those who have diabetes or prediabetes. Stress causes our bodies to release adrenaline and cortisol, two substances that can increase blood sugar. Those who already have trouble keeping their blood sugar levels consistent may find this to be especially difficult. Thus, using stress-reduction strategies is essential to controlling blood sugar levels. The following are some practical stress-reduction methods that are especially useful for blood sugar stabilization:

1. Engage in deep breathing exercises: These techniques assist in triggering the body's relaxation response and reducing tension. You can lessen stress and the generation of cortisol by inhaling deeply from your nose and exhaling slowly through your mouth. This will help to normalize blood sugar levels.

2. Work out frequently: Research has shown that physical activity reduces stress. Frequent exercise lowers stress and enhances general wellbeing in addition to improving insulin sensitivity, which helps control blood sugar levels. Walking, swimming, yoga, dancing, and other enjoyable activities can help lower stress and maintain stable blood sugar levels.

3. Engage in mindfulness and meditation: These practices can aid in stress reduction and the enhancement of emotional health. You can reduce stress and enhance blood sugar regulation by concentrating on the here and now and paying attention to your thoughts without passing judgment. In particular, stress management and blood sugar stability can be achieved with the use of meditation techniques such as guided imagery or body scans.

4. Get enough good sleep: Stress and blood sugar regulation both depend on getting enough sleep. Chronic sleep deprivation can raise cortisol levels, which in turn can raise blood sugar. To encourage improved sleep hygiene, aim for seven to eight hours of high-quality sleep every night, set up a reliable sleep schedule, and design a sleep-friendly atmosphere.

5. Take part in stress-relieving activities: Taking part in enjoyable and relaxing activities might help you manage stress and keep your blood sugar levels stable. Hobbies, spending time with loved ones, reading, listening to music, and taking soothing baths are a few examples. Make relaxing activities a regular part of your schedule by finding ones that you enjoy.

6. Seek assistance: Having a support network can be beneficial when controlling blood sugar and stress. Speak with dependable family members, friends, or support groups for guidance and assistance in overcoming obstacles. Gaining further knowledge of stress-reduction and coping mechanisms can also be facilitated by seeking professional assistance, such as therapy or counseling.

7. Make self-care a priority: Maintaining stable blood sugar levels and stress management depend on you taking care of yourself. Allocate time for pursuits that enhance your mental, emotional, and physical health. This could be maintaining a healthy diet, managing diabetes well, going outside, reading inspirational literature, or reflecting on oneself.

In summary, stress management is essential for people with diabetes or prediabetes to keep their blood sugar levels steady. Deep breathing, consistent exercise, mindfulness, and getting enough sleep are just a few of the stress-reduction strategies that can help lower stress levels and improve blood sugar regulation. Make stress management a top priority in your everyday activities, and seek the individualized advice of medical professionals.

Although these stress-reduction methods can help stabilize blood sugar levels, it's still advisable to speak with a healthcare provider for specific advice and recommendations tailored to your unique situation and medical condition.

The Importance of Quality Sleep in Blood Sugar Control,

Getting enough sleep is crucial for maintaining general health and controlling blood sugar levels. For people who currently have diabetes or are at risk of getting it, it is extremely important. Having a healthy sleep schedule is essential for controlling blood sugar levels.

Getting enough sleep has a major impact on hormone control, especially when it comes to cortisol and insulin. Insulin aids in the body's utilization and maintenance of optimum glucose levels. On the other hand, insufficient or disturbed sleep can cause insulin resistance, which impairs the body's ability to react appropriately to insulin.

This may lead to higher blood sugar levels and a higher chance of getting diabetes. Inadequate sleep can also result in high cortisol levels, which can worsen insulin resistance.

Additionally, getting enough sleep reduces the risk of obesity and aids in weight management. Lack of sleep throws off the hormone balance that controls appetite and satiety, which increases hunger. The body's capacity to digest carbohydrates is impacted by sleep deprivation, which may lead to decreased glucose tolerance and even elevated blood sugar levels.

Good sleep has an impact on mental and emotional health in addition to hormone management. Insufficient sleep has been linked to elevated levels of stress, worry, and depression. These factors can complicate the task of properly managing diabetes and controlling blood sugar levels.

Multiple measures can be employed to guarantee optimal blood sugar regulation and promote quality sleep:

1. Keep a regular sleep schedule: Having regular bedtimes and wake-up hours encourages healthy sleep habits by assisting the body's internal clock.

2. Create a sleep-friendly environment: To encourage unwinding and restful sleep, make your bedroom cozy, dark, and quiet. Reduce your exposure to electronic screens and harsh lights to improve the quality of your sleep.

3. Use relaxation methods: You can lower your stress levels before bed and improve your quality of sleep by using methods like deep breathing exercises, meditation, or a calming bedtime ritual.

4. Exercise on a regular basis: Frequent exercise during the day can enhance the quality of your sleep, encourage relaxation, and assist with blood sugar regulation.

5. Limit stimulants: To avoid sleep problems, cut back on your caffeine intake, particularly in the afternoon and evening.

In summary, getting enough sleep is essential for preserving blood sugar regulation and general health. People can control their weight, lower their stress levels, manage their hormones, and enhance their overall wellbeing by making good sleep habits a priority. Prioritizing sleep is crucial for optimal blood sugar control and diabetes treatment, along with other healthy lifestyle choices.

Chapter 8: Troubleshooting and Overcoming Challenges

Sustaining appropriate blood glucose levels is critical for general health, particularly for those with diabetes and other medical disorders. Although controlling blood sugar levels using a blood sugar diet is an efficient strategy, it is not without its difficulties. In order to successfully control blood sugar levels with dietary modifications over the long term, it is imperative to troubleshoot and overcome these obstacles.

Making the adjustment to a new eating pattern is one of the frequent problems people following a blood sugar diet solution encounter. Changing eating habits and including new items in regular meals can be daunting at first. It is possible to overcome this obstacle by beginning with modest, doable measures. A smoother transition can be achieved by including new foods and recipes into one's diet gradually. A nutritionist or dietitian with expertise in blood sugar management can also be a great resource for helping you comprehend and successfully apply the required dietary adjustments.

In a blood sugar diet, controlling cravings for harmful, high-sugar foods is another difficulty. In the beginning while the body is still getting used to eating less sugar, these cravings can be very strong and challenging to ignore. To conquer this obstacle, one must combine determination with healthful substitutes. You can assist satiate cravings while following the dietary rules by substituting fruits for sugary treats or using natural sweeteners like stevia. Cravings may become less intense over time as the body gets used to consuming less sugar, which will make it simpler to avoid bad choices.

Organizing and preparing meals might be difficult while following a blood sugar diet. Because it might be difficult to find time for meal planning and preparation due to busy schedules, people may rely more on processed meals or unhealthy takeout.   This difficulty can be met, though, with careful preparation and coordination. Meal planning, grocery shopping, and meal preparation can be made much simpler by setting aside a specified time each week. Meal planning on the weekends can save a lot of time and guarantee that healthier options are accessible by dedicating a few hours of your weekend to the task.

An additional critical component of blood sugar management is the monitoring of blood sugar levels and the dietary modifications made in response. Finding the right ratio of fats, proteins, and carbohydrates for the unique requirements of each person can be difficult, though. This difficulty can be overcome by routinely checking blood sugar levels and speaking with medical experts to determine individualized dietary needs. Based on individual reactions and long-term blood sugar level measurements, modifications to the blood sugar diet plan might be necessary.

Last but not least, a blood sugar diet solution's ability to face and overcome obstacles depends greatly on the support of friends and family. Having a strong support system around oneself can offer inspiration, responsibility, and even fresh ideas for dishes and way of life adjustments. Participating in blood sugar management support groups or online forums can be a great way to get advice and motivation.

In conclusion, although implementing a blood sugar diet has its share of difficulties, these may be resolved with perseverance, resolve, and the appropriate strategy. People can successfully manage their blood sugar levels and lead healthier lives by breaking the transition down into manageable steps, finding healthy alternatives to fight cravings, embracing meal planning and preparation, actively monitoring blood sugar levels, and asking for support from loved ones.

Dealing with Cravings and Emotional Eating

Handling Diabetes's Cravings and Emotional Eating

A nutritious diet is just one of the many lifestyle adjustments needed to manage diabetes. But maintaining a strict diet can be difficult at times, particularly when cravings and emotional eating triggers are present. Dealing with these situations effectively requires an understanding of the connection between emotions, appetites, and diabetes. People with diabetes can maintain stable blood sugar levels and general well-being by adopting techniques to control cravings and emotional eating.

1. Determine the triggers:

Identifying the causes that cause cravings and emotional eating is the first step towards controlling them. It can be a particular food item, boredom, tension, or grief. To better understand your own triggers, observe when and why cravings occur.

2. Get Yourself Amused:

When a craving occurs, consider diverting your focus with other tasks to help you pass the time. Take a walk, give someone a call, read a book, engage in a hobby, or do anything else that will divert your attention from food.

3. Make smart meal plans:

Make sure your meals contain a range of nutrients, including whole grains, lean proteins, and an abundance of fruits and vegetables. This will lessen the likelihood that you will feel starved or have strong desires, and it will help to guarantee that you are eating a balanced diet.

4. Make mindful food choices:

Emotional eating frequently happens when we eat without thinking and ignore our hunger or fullness signs. By chewing carefully, enjoying each bite, and focusing on the flavors, textures, and aromas of the meal, you can try to practice mindful eating. This will assist you in distinguishing between eating for emotional reasons and when you are actually hungry.

5. Look for assistance:

Managing emotional eating can be greatly improved by having a support system. Speak with your loved ones, close friends, or a support group for motivation and guidance. Talk to them about your challenges, achievements, and tactics; they might have insightful stories to share.

6. Look for healthier substitutes:

If there are certain meals that you crave often, look for healthier substitutes that can satiate your cravings without affecting your blood sugar regulation. For instance, include naturally sweet fruits in your diet if you have a sweet tooth. Baked veggie chips or air-popped popcorn are good options if you're craving salty food.

7. Control Your Stress:

A frequent cause of emotional eating is stress. Learn effective coping mechanisms for stress, such as deep breathing exercises, frequent exercise, meditation, or hobbies. Reducing stress might lessen the chance that you'll go for food to comfort yourself.

8. Seek Expert Assistance:

You might find it helpful to consult with a licensed dietitian, therapist, or diabetes educator if you are having trouble managing your cravings and emotional eating on your own. These experts can offer you individualized advice and assistance in creating coping mechanisms that are tailored to your needs.

Recall that controlling cravings and emotional eating takes time. Try not to be too hard on yourself when mistakes are made. It takes perseverance to manage diabetes, but you can eventually form better habits that put your health first.

Strategies for Dining Out and Social Situations

For those with diabetes or other diseases requiring blood glucose control, controlling blood sugar levels is crucial.

Social gatherings and eating out can be difficult because they frequently feature rich, high-carbohydrate foods and beverages. However, these events can be enjoyed without having a detrimental effect on blood sugar levels if appropriate planning and procedures are used.

The following are some practical methods for controlling blood sugar when dining out and interacting with others:

1. Pick your restaurant wisely: Give top priority to establishments that provide a range of healthful options, such as vegetables, whole grains, lean proteins, and balanced meals. Nowadays, a lot of businesses offer nutrition information online, which is useful for making well-informed food decisions.

2. Make a plan in advance: Before dining out, if at all possible, go over the menu. Seek alternatives that meet your dietary requirements. This preparation frees you from the menu's alluring descriptions and other influences so that you can make a thoughtful choice.

3. Regulate portion sizes: Restaurants frequently serve large portions, which can cause overindulgence and blood sugar increases. If you are dining with someone, think about splitting an appetizer or main course, or ask the waitress to pack half of your meal to go before it is served.

4. Make drinking water a priority. Be sure to stay hydrated by sipping water at every meal. This can help avoid overeating and aid with digestion in addition to relieving thirst. Sugary drinks, such as soda, mixed drinks, and fruit juices, should be avoided or consumed in moderation because they can quickly raise blood sugar levels.

5. Mindful eating: Take your time and enjoy your meal. Give each bite some time to really enjoy its flavors, textures, and fragrances. By allowing your body more time to detect fullness, eating slowly can help you avoid overindulging and maintain stable blood sugar levels.

6. Change your order: Don't be afraid to ask the server to substitute an item or adjust the recipe to suit your preferences. For instance, you could ask for a salad as a side dish rather than pasta or fries.

7. Be mindful of cooking techniques: Choose baked, roasted, or grilling foods instead of frying or breading them, as they are typically healthier options. These cooking techniques frequently lower the meal's total fat and calorie intake.

8. Use caution when adding extras and condiments: Dressings, sauces, and toppings can have sugars or fats that shouldn't be there. To manage the quantity you use, ask for dressings and sauces on the side or ask for healthy substitutes like vinegar or olive oil.

9. Tell your friends and family about your food limits and health objectives. They will be able to respect and support your decisions, and it might even affect how they choose to eat.

10. Bring snacks or glucose pills: It's always convenient to have a snack or glucose tablets on hand to promptly address any symptoms of low blood sugar, especially if you're unclear of the meal options available or anticipate potential delays.

To guarantee that your meal plan and methods are in line with your unique health demands and medications, don't forget to coordinate them with your healthcare physician or registered dietitian.

Through the implementation of these tactics, people can effectively regulate their blood sugar levels when dining out and in social settings, all the while indulging in delectable meals and engaging with friends and family.

Plateaus and How to Break Through Them

When it comes to controlling blood sugar, plateaus are a frequent and annoying phenomenon. Hitting a plateau can impede your progress and make it more challenging to meet your health objectives, regardless of whether you have diabetes or are just attempting to maintain stable blood sugar levels. But you may overcome these plateaus and improve your blood sugar control with the correct techniques and persistence.

Insulin resistance is one of the main causes of blood sugar plateaus. The pancreas secretes the hormone insulin, which aids in controlling blood sugar levels. Blood sugar levels rise when the body develops a resistance to insulin, which makes it more difficult for glucose to enter the cells. Numerous factors, including obesity, a sedentary lifestyle, a bad diet, or specific medical disorders, may contribute to this insulin resistance.

It's critical to treat the underlying cause of insulin resistance in order to overcome the plateau. The following tactics may be useful:

1. Make dietary adjustments: Put your attention on eating a well-balanced diet rich in whole foods including fruits, vegetables, lean meats, and whole grains. Steer clear of processed foods, sugary beverages, and meals high in carbohydrates. To avoid blood sugar spikes, think about cutting back on your carbohydrate intake and choosing foods with a low glycemic index.

2. Exercise on a regular basis: Controlling blood sugar levels requires frequent exercise. Exercises like swimming, cycling, strength training, or brisk walking can help overcome the plateau and enhance insulin sensitivity. Try to get in at least 150 minutes a week of moderate-to-intense activity.

3. Keep an eye on your medication: Speak with your doctor to make sure the dosage you're taking is right for your present health. To help control your blood sugar levels, they can suggest experimenting with new drugs or modifying dosages.

4. Control your stress levels: Prolonged stress has been linked to high blood sugar. Include stress-reduction strategies such as yoga, meditation, deep breathing exercises, or relaxing hobbies. Lowering stress levels has a beneficial effect on blood sugar regulation.

5. Get enough sleep: Sleep deprivation might alter insulin sensitivity and cause blood sugar swings. For the best possible blood sugar regulation, try to get seven or eight hours of good sleep every night.

6. Track and monitor your blood sugar levels: Measure your blood sugar on a regular basis to look for trends and modify your plan of action accordingly. You can better understand how your body reacts to specific foods, activities, or drugs by doing frequent monitoring.

7. Look for assistance: Participating in a support group or getting advice from a certified dietitian or diabetes educator can offer insightful information and inspiration to break through plateaus. They can help you customize your methods to meet your unique demands and provide you with individualized advice.

Recall that overcoming blood sugar plateaus requires patience and time. Positive outcomes will eventually come from being proactive and consistent with your lifestyle modifications. You may restore control over your blood sugar levels and improve your general health by addressing the underlying reasons for insulin resistance, adopting healthier lifestyle choices, and consulting a medical expert.

Chapter 9:
Monitoring and Tracking Blood Sugar Levels

Blood sugar levels should be tracked and monitored closely by those who have diabetes or are at risk of getting it. It is an essential tool for both keeping well and controlling the illness. By monitoring their blood sugar, people can learn how their bodies react to various stimulants, diets, activities, and stress levels. This knowledge empowers them to make well-informed decisions and modify their lifestyle.

Blood sugar levels can be effectively monitored using a number of techniques, such as laboratory tests, continuous glucose monitoring (CGM), and self-monitoring blood glucose (SMBG).

1. Blood glucose self-monitoring (SBG):
A finger-stick blood glucose meter is used in SMBG to measure blood sugar levels at different times of the day. Typically, the procedure is using a lancet to pierce the fingertip in order to draw blood, putting the blood on a test strip, and then placing the strip into the meter to read it. Users can quickly and easily monitor their blood sugar levels with SMBG, which is readily available. Finding patterns—such as elevated or lowered blood sugar

during particular hours of the day or following particular meals—is helpful. For those who need insulin to control their diabetes, SMBG is very helpful because they must modify their insulin dosage according to their blood sugar levels.

2. Insulin Gene Continuum (IGC):

CGM systems are gadgets that give users access to real-time data on their blood sugar levels day and night. A tiny sensor that detects the amount of glucose in the interstitial fluid is placed beneath the skin, generally in the arm or belly. A receiver or smartphone receives the data wirelessly from the sensor, allowing users to examine their glucose readings, trends, and receive alarms for high or low levels. Since CGM devices take data every few minutes, they offer a more complete picture of blood sugar levels. This makes it easier for people to see trends and comprehend how their blood sugar levels change during the day, including when they sleep. Those who have recurrent hypoglycemic episodes or have trouble identifying the symptoms of hypoglycemia would benefit most from CGM.

3. Exams in a lab:

Drawing blood and sending it to a lab for analysis is known as laboratory testing. This technique confirms glucose anomalies found by SMBG or CGM and yields precise and accurate findings. Glycated hemoglobin

(HbA1c), the oral glucose tolerance test (OGTT), and fasting plasma glucose (FPG) are examples of laboratory testing. Following a minimum of eight hours of fasting, FPG measures blood glucose. Once a high-glucose beverage is consumed, the body's reaction to glucose is evaluated using the OGTT. The average blood glucose levels over the previous two to three months are shown by the HbA1c. Diagnosing diabetes and tracking long-term blood sugar control require laboratory testing. Whatever the technique, regular blood sugar testing and monitoring offer important insights into a person's overall management of their diabetes. People can maintain ideal blood sugar management by making educated decisions about their diet, exercise routine, medicine, and other lifestyle choices by routinely testing their glucose levels. The right target glucose range and monitoring strategy should be chosen in consultation with healthcare providers in order to take into account each person's needs and objectives.

Tools and Techniques for Blood Sugar Monitoring

A vital component of controlling diabetes and preserving ideal blood glucose levels is blood sugar monitoring. This procedure has been transformed by the availability of numerous instruments and methods, enabling people to conveniently and accurately check their blood sugar levels from the comfort of their homes. Here are a few methods and instruments for checking blood sugar that are often used:

1. Glucometer: A portable instrument for determining blood sugar levels is a glucometer. It takes a tiny amount of blood, usually drawn using a lancet and administered to a test strip that is placed inside the glucometer. In a matter of seconds, the gadget offers a computerized blood sugar readout. Glucometers are lightweight and convenient to carry about for routine observation.

2. Continuous Glucose Monitoring (CGM) System: CGM systems use a tiny sensor that is usually placed on the belly and placed under the skin. The sensor wirelessly sends the data to a receiver or smartphone app after continually measuring the interstitial fluid's glucose levels. Real-time blood sugar measurements from CGM devices are available, along with trends and alarms for elevated or lowered glucose levels.

3. Flash Glucose Monitoring (FGM) System: FGM systems function similarly to CGM systems but don't need to be calibrated with frequent finger pricks. Instead, glucose levels and historical trends are obtained by scanning the sensor with a reader device or smartphone app. People who hate repeated finger pricks frequently favor FGM systems.

4. Insulin Pump: A lot of insulin pumps these days come with CGM integration, enabling both insulin delivery and continuous glucose monitoring. Through the use of a tiny catheter that is put beneath the skin and attached to the pump, these devices administer insulin. For those who need insulin therapy, the combination of glucose monitoring and insulin delivery makes diabetes control easier.

5. Mobile Apps: These days, people frequently use mobile applications to check their blood sugar levels. Meals, exercise, blood glucose levels, medications, and other pertinent data can all be tracked using these apps. Additionally, some apps include capabilities like personalized suggestions, glucose trend analysis, and data sharing with medical specialists.

6. Remote Monitoring: Medical personnel can remotely check on patients' blood sugar levels thanks to the use of remote monitoring devices, which are frequently employed in clinical settings. Patients can upload their blood glucose readings using these devices, and healthcare professionals can access them for analysis and necessary intervention. Plans for managing diabetes can be adjusted with the help of useful information obtained from remote monitoring.

7. Data Management Software: A lot of blood glucose monitors include data management software, which enables users to download and examine their findings. Graphs, charts, and reports are frequently provided by these software packages to assist users in understanding patterns and trends in their blood sugar levels over time.

People with diabetes can make more informed decisions regarding their diet, exercise routine, medicine, and overall diabetes management with the use of efficient blood sugar monitoring equipment and approaches. In order to avoid difficulties and maintain a healthy lifestyle, regular blood sugar analysis and monitoring are essential. It is crucial to speak with medical professionals to find the best blood sugar monitoring equipment and methods for your particular needs and situation.

Interpreting Blood Sugar Readings and Making Adjustments

Understanding blood sugar readings is essential to properly controlling diabetes. By being aware of these readings, people can maintain ideal blood sugar levels by modifying their food, taking their medications, and engaging in general health activities. The following are important things to keep in mind while analyzing blood sugar values and adjusting as necessary:

1. Understand the target range: It's critical to understand the target blood sugar range that your doctor has prescribed. For most diabetics, a postprandial (after-meal) blood sugar level of less than 180 mg/dL and a fasting blood sugar level of 80–130 mg/dL are considered to be within the normal range. These goals, however, may change based on variables like age, diabetes type, and general health.

2. Check your readings frequently: Using a glucose meter or continuous glucose monitoring (CGM) system, it's imperative to frequently check your blood sugar levels. Frequent observation makes it easier to spot patterns and trends, which empowers you to make wise corrections. To obtain precise information about your blood sugar levels throughout the day, try to stick to a regular testing routine.

3. Recognize the impact of meals and exercise: Eating habits and exercise can have a significant impact on blood sugar levels. Examining blood sugar measurements in conjunction with information about meals eaten and exercise done can yield insightful results. This helps you make the required modifications to maintain stable readings by enabling you to recognize how certain diets or exercise regimens may affect your blood sugar levels.

4. Identify the signs of high and low blood sugar:
Hyperglycemia, or elevated blood sugar, is characterized
by increased thirst, frequent urination, lethargy, impaired
vision, and sluggish wound healing. Hypoglycemia, or
low blood sugar, can cause symptoms including
trembling, lightheadedness, confusion, sweating, and an
accelerated heartbeat. By being aware of these symptoms
and connecting them to particular blood sugar levels,
you can take preventive measures to avoid
consequences.

5. Modifying insulin and medication dosages: You can
ascertain whether adjustments to insulin or medication
dosages are required by interpreting blood sugar
measurements. Adopting lifestyle alterations such as
dietary adjustments or increasing physical exercise can
occasionally assist maintain stable blood sugar levels
without the need to adjust medications. However, before
adjusting your medicine or insulin dosage, it is
imperative that you speak with your healthcare
professional.

6. Seek expert advice: Interpreting blood sugar readings
can be difficult, particularly for those who are newly
diagnosed or who fluctuate frequently. Consulting a
dietitian, diabetic educator, or medical professional can
offer priceless assistance. They can assist you in
identifying trends in your readings, modifying as

necessary, and creating individualized plans to more effectively control your blood sugar levels.

Keep in mind that each person has a different blood sugar reaction, so what works for one person might not work for another. Effective diabetes care requires regular monitoring, pattern analysis, and professional advice. Diabetes can be better managed by people with the disease by regularly making the required modifications and properly evaluating blood sugar readings. This can lead to an improvement in overall health and well-being.

Chapter 10:
Long-Term Maintenance and Support

For those with diabetes, controlling blood sugar levels requires ongoing care and assistance. Maintaining blood sugar management is essential for avoiding diabetes-related consequences such as kidney damage, nerve damage, eyesight issues, and cardiovascular disease. Thus, to guarantee stable blood sugar levels and general health, a thorough plan for long-term maintenance and support must be established.

Adopting a healthy lifestyle is a crucial element of long-term maintenance and support. This entails maintaining a healthy weight, getting regular exercise, eating a balanced diet, and managing stress. Blood sugar levels can be regulated with a diet high in fruits, vegetables, whole grains, lean meats, and healthy fats. Limiting sugar-filled foods, processed carbs, and unhealthy fats is also crucial because they can raise blood sugar levels.

Blood sugar control is significantly influenced by regular physical activity. Exercises like swimming, cycling, jogging, and walking increase insulin sensitivity and assist the body in using glucose for energy. It is advised to perform strength training activities two to three times a week in addition to at least 150 minutes of moderate-intensity aerobic activity per week.

Maintaining a healthy weight is also essential for long-term blood sugar regulation. Sustaining a healthy weight or, if needed, losing weight can enhance insulin resistance and lower the chance of complications from diabetes. This can be accomplished by combining a diet low in calories with frequent physical activity.

Regular blood sugar monitoring is another crucial component of long-term care. By monitoring blood sugar levels, people can spot patterns and trends and alter their diet, exercise routine, or medication schedule as needed. A continuous glucose monitoring (CGM) system, which offers real-time data on blood sugar levels throughout the day, or a blood glucose meter can be used for this.

For long-term assistance, routine visits to medical specialists are essential. These specialists include diabetes educators, endocrinologists, and primary care physicians. These experts can answer any queries or concerns people may have regarding their blood sugar control in addition to offering advice on medication administration and lifestyle changes. They are also capable of offering the proper interventions and keeping an eye out for any possible difficulties.

Furthermore, emotional well-being should be taken into account for long-term maintenance and assistance. Diabetes can occasionally be emotionally taxing and hard to live with. Seeking assistance from loved ones, friends, and support groups is crucial since they can offer inspiration, empathy, and useful guidance. Furthermore, practicing stress-reduction methods like deep breathing exercises, meditation, or taking up enjoyable hobbies and pastimes can help lower stress levels, which can improve blood sugar regulation.

In conclusion, in order for people with diabetes to effectively control their blood sugar levels and stop problems from developing, long-term maintenance and assistance are essential. An all-encompassing strategy that incorporates leading a healthy lifestyle, frequent monitoring, medical appointments, and mental health can result in better long-term blood sugar regulation and general quality of life.

Strategies for Maintaining Blood Sugar Stability

The following tactics can be used to keep blood sugar stable:

1. Consume a diet that is well-balanced: Make sure your meals contain a variety of proteins, carbs, and healthy fats. Steer clear of processed meals and refined sweets in favor of whole foods.

2. Pay attention to portion sizes: To prevent overindulging or consuming too many carbohydrates, pay attention to portion proportions.

3. Consume regular meals and snacks: Maintain a regular eating routine by distributing meals and snacks equally throughout the day. This lessens the chance of blood sugar crashes and spikes.

- Select meals with a low glycemic index (GI) to help regulate blood sugar levels. GI-rated foods release sugar into the bloodstream more gradually. Lean proteins, non-starchy veggies, lentils, and whole grains are your best options.

- Consume a lot of foods high in fiber, such as whole grains, beans, fruits, and vegetables. Fiber increases satiety by delaying the bloodstream's absorption of sugar.

4. Remain hydrated: To prevent dehydration, which can impact blood sugar levels, drink adequate water throughout the day. Drink less sugar-filled beverages and more water, herbal tea, or unsweetened tea.

5. Exercise on a regular basis: Perform strength and aerobic training exercises on a regular basis. Increased insulin sensitivity from physical activity enables more effective blood sugar management.

6. Get enough rest: Try to get seven to eight hours of good sleep every night. Hormones that control blood sugar might be upset by sleep deprivation, which can result in instability.

7. Stress management: Look for healthy methods to reduce stress, such mindfulness, yoga, deep breathing techniques, or taking up a hobby. Blood sugar levels can be impacted by ongoing stress.

8. Monitor blood sugar levels: If you have diabetes or are at risk for high blood sugar, check your blood sugar levels on a regular basis with a glucose meter. This enables you to monitor your development and make the required dietary and lifestyle changes.

9. Adherence to medicine: If your doctor has recommended medication to control your blood sugar, take it exactly as instructed. As advised, get frequent check-ups afterward.

10. Consult a medical professional: Speak with a healthcare physician or certified dietitian who specializes in managing blood sugar levels or diabetes. They may offer you individualized advice, teach you about healthy eating, and assist in making a plan that is specific to your requirements.

11. Take into account glycemic load: This is another factor to think about besides the glycemic index. It considers the amount and quality of carbohydrates a food contains. This can give a more realistic impression of the potential effects of a food on blood sugar levels.

12. Limit alcohol intake: Due to its ability to promote blood sugar swings, alcohol should be avoided or consumed in moderation.

13. Become knowledgeable: Keep up to date on blood sugar control techniques and arm yourself with information. Learn about the effects of food on blood sugar levels, portion sizes, and nutrition.

Recall that seeing a healthcare provider is crucial, particularly if you have a medical condition like diabetes. They can offer tailored counsel and direction according to your particular requirements.

Seeking Professional Guidance and Support

Seeking Expert Advice and Assistance: Making the Transition to Personal Development and Self-Empowerment

Today's world is fast-paced and complex, making it easy to feel overwhelmed at times when faced with obstacles.

Seeking professional advice and support may be a significant step towards achieving personal growth and empowerment, regardless of the personal or professional concerns we are facing, such as depression, anxiety, relationship problems, or work challenges.

A lot of people tend to undervalue the benefits that they might receive from getting professional assistance. Despite what many people think, asking for help doesn't indicate weakness; rather, it shows strength and a desire to better oneself. It requires bravery to admit when we need help and to take the required actions to get it.

There are many different kinds of professionals who can offer guidance: therapists, psychologists, counselors, life coaches, and career advisors. These professionals are well-versed in their disciplines and prepared to assist people in facing obstacles head-on, gaining understanding of their own thoughts and actions, and creating useful coping strategies.

Having the freedom to freely and honestly express oneself is one of the most significant benefits of getting expert advice and assistance. Many people find it difficult to be vulnerable with friends and family because they are afraid of being judged or because they don't fully comprehend the complexity of their situation. Professional counselors, on the other hand, offer a secure and judgment-free setting where people can openly and honestly share their feelings.

Therapists can assist clients in exploring their thoughts, feelings, and behavioural patterns using various therapy procedures and strategies. They promote introspection, which aids people in comprehending who they are and the elements influencing their problems. People can become more self-aware and recognize possible areas for development and progress by doing this.

Furthermore, obtaining expert advice and assistance can provide people with the abilities and resources needed to successfully address their obstacles. Experts provide individualized guidance and research-backed treatment approaches that enable people to overcome challenges, control their stress, and adopt more positive thought and behaviour patterns. Better decision-making, stronger bonds with others, greater self-assurance, and an elevated sense of general wellbeing can all result from this assistance.

It is crucial to keep in mind that asking for help and advice from professionals is a proactive move towards personal development. It is not just for emergencies; it may also be quite helpful in averting future issues and improving general well-being. By making an investment in our mental and emotional health through expert counseling, we show that we value our mental and emotional health and strengthen our ability to overcome obstacles in the future.

In conclusion, make the courageous and empowering decision to seek expert advice and assistance. It enables people to become more self-aware, take a proactive stance towards their own development, and create useful coping mechanisms. People can overcome obstacles, enhance their emotional health, and develop a more purposeful and independent existence by consulting specialists. Recall that asking for assistance is never a sign of weakness but rather of strength and a desire to enjoy life to the fullest.

Celebrating Success and Staying Motivated

Showcasing Achievement and Maintaining Drive with a Blood Sugar Diet Approach

Making the decision to change to a healthier lifestyle might be difficult, but success is possible if you have the correct attitude and strategy. Adhering to a blood sugar diet plan improves general well being in addition to aiding in weight loss. Maintaining your motivation and acknowledging your accomplishments along the way are essential components of a well-mapped out plan for achieving your fitness and health objectives.

Honoring accomplishments is a crucial step in the procedure. You'll be more inspired and driven to reach your next objective if you take the time to acknowledge and celebrate your accomplishments.

Celebrating these victories is crucial, whether they involve hitting a blood sugar target, dropping a specified amount of weight, or simply getting through a difficult week. Select incentives that support your health objectives, such as purchasing new sports attire, getting a soothing massage, or indulging in a tasty but nutritious dinner. Celebrating your accomplishments encourages you to keep up the good work you are doing in your life and also helps to lift your spirits.

As with any lifestyle adjustment, there will inevitably be times when motivation falters. You can, however, prevent reverting to your old behaviors by implementing techniques for maintaining motivation. Here are some pointers to keep you on course:

1. Establish reachable and realistic goals: Divide your overarching goals into more manageable subgoals. This will maintain motivation and facilitate the tracking of progress.

2. Surround yourself with support: You can get the accountability and support you need to stay motivated by joining a group of like-minded people or by asking a coach or nutritionist for advice. To create an environment that is upbeat and supportive, share your triumphs, difficulties, and advice with others.

3. Keep a journal: Writing down your experiences—both the successes and the setbacks—can act as a strong reflection of your development and a source of inspiration when things get tough.

4. Find motivation: Look for testimonials from people who have successfully adhered to a blood sugar diet plan. Learning about their successes and the advantages they have enjoyed can bolster your confidence in the program and increase your enthusiasm.

5. Make it fun: Look for methods to add enjoyment to your new eating habits by experimenting with different foods, trying out new recipes, and developing an appreciation for the nutrients and flavors that help you achieve your health objectives.

6. Keep track of your progress: Seeing your development might serve as inspiration. Maintaining a regular log of metrics like weight, blood sugar, and body measurements will help you stay motivated to stick with your blood sugar diet plan by giving you concrete proof of your progress.

Recall that maintaining motivation requires work. It's
common to have periods of uncertainty or
disappointment, but it's critical to keep in mind the
motivation behind your initial efforts and the progress
you have already achieved. Your resolve to stick with
your blood sugar diet solution route to better health and
wellbeing will be strengthened by acknowledging your
accomplishments and developing techniques for
maintaining motivation.

Conclusion

In summary, the blood sugar diet solution presents a viable strategy for controlling and enhancing blood sugar levels, controlling weight, and enhancing general health. This diet attempts to lower inflammation, stabilize blood sugar levels, and encourage weight loss by emphasizing low-carb and Mediterranean-style meals, frequent exercise, and intermittent fasting. This diet has been shown to enhance insulin sensitivity, lower the risk of chronic illnesses, and boost energy levels. Furthermore, in the long run, this diet is easily adaptable and sustainable for one's lifestyle. Before beginning any new diet or fitness regimen, it is crucial to speak with a healthcare provider, especially for people who have specific dietary requirements or pre-existing medical conditions. All things considered, the blood sugar diet solution offers a workable and efficient way for people to better control their blood sugar levels and reach their ideal health.

Achieving Balanced Blood Sugar and Improved Wellbeing

In conclusion, achieving balanced blood sugar levels is crucial for overall health and well-being. Maintaining a balanced blood sugar level not only benefits individuals with diabetes but also has numerous positive effects on overall health. It can improve energy levels, mood, mental clarity, and weight management. Through lifestyle changes such as regular physical activity, healthy eating habits, stress management, and adequate sleep, individuals can achieve balanced blood sugar levels and improve their overall well-being. Additionally, it is important to monitor blood sugar levels regularly and consult a healthcare professional for personalized advice and guidance. By prioritizing balanced blood sugar, individuals can experience an enhanced quality of life and reduce the risk of developing chronic conditions.